100 Questions & Answers About Leukemia

Third Edition

Edward D. Ball, MD

Professor of Medicine
Chief, Division of Blood and Marrow Transplantation
Moores Cancer Center, University of California at San Diego
La Jolla, CA

Alex Kagan

San Diego, CA

JONES & BARTLETT
L E A R N I N G

World Headquarters
Jones & Bartlett Learning
5 Wall Street
Burlington, MA 01803
978-443-5000
info@jblearning.com
www.jblearning.com

Jones & Bartlett Learning books and products are available through most bookstores and online booksellers.
To contact Jones & Bartlett Learning directly, call 800-832-0034, fax 978-443-8000, or visit our website,
www.jblearning.com.

Substantial discounts on bulk quantities of Jones & Bartlett Learning publications are available to corporations,
professional associations, and other qualified organizations. For details and specific discount information, contact
the special sales department at Jones & Bartlett Learning via the above contact information or send an email to
specialsales@jblearning.com.

100 Questions & Answers About Leukemia, Third Edition, is an independent publication and has not been authorized,
sponsored, or otherwise approved by the owners of the trademarks or service marks referenced in this product.

Some images in this book feature models. These models do not necessarily endorse, represent, or participate in the
activities represented in the images.

The authors, editor, and publisher have made every effort to provide accurate information. However, they are not
responsible for errors, omissions, or for any outcomes related to the use of the contents of this book and take no
responsibility for the use of the products and procedures described. Treatments and side effects described in this book
may not be applicable to all people; likewise, some people may require a dose or experience a side effect that is not
described herein. Drugs and medical devices are discussed that may have limited availability controlled by the Food
and Drug Administration (FDA) for use only in a research study or clinical trial. Research, clinical practice, and
government regulations often change the accepted standard in this field. When consideration is being given to use
of any drug in the clinical setting, the health care provider or reader is responsible for determining FDA status of the
drug, reading the package insert, and reviewing prescribing information for the most up-to-date recommendations
on dose, precautions, and contraindications, and determining the appropriate usage for the product. This is especially
important in the case of drugs that are new or seldom used.

Production Credits
Executive Publisher: Christopher Davis
Associate Editor: Laura Burns
Production Editor: Dan Stone
Senior Manufacturing and Inventory Control
   Supervisor: Amy Bacus
Marketing Manager, Medicine: Rebecca Rockel
Composition: Abella Publishing Services, LLC

Cover Design: Carolyn Downer
Cover Credits: Top: © *iStockphoto/Thinkstock;* Bottom
   Left: © *Laurence Mouton/PhotoAlto/Jupiterimages;*
   Bottom Right: © *Siri Stafford/Lifesize/Thinkstock*
Printing and Binding: Edwards Brothers Malloy
Cover Printing: Edwards Brothers Malloy

Library of Congress Cataloging-in-Publication Data
Ball, Edward D. (Edward David), 1950-
  100 questions & answers about leukemia / Edward D. Ball, Alex Kagan. — 3rd ed.
    p. cm.
  Includes index.
  ISBN 978-1-4496-6583-8
1. Leukemia—Popular works. 2. Leukemia—Miscellanea. I. Kagan, Alex. II. Title. III. Title: 100 questions and
answers about leukemia. IV. Title: One hundred questions and answers about leukemia.
  RC643.B355 2013
  616.99'419--dc23
                  2012010529
6048

Printed in the United States of America
16 15 14 13 12   10 9 8 7 6 5 4 3 2 1

CONTENTS

The diagnosis "leukemia" strikes fear into the heart of a patient. Indeed, the diagnosis of leukemia implies profound changes for the patient and his/her loved ones. Many spheres of life will be greatly impacted, including relationships with others, view of self, ability to work, sexual function, as well as the length of life itself. Worrying about all these aspects of self is an enormous challenge for an individual and his/her family. One critical way to deal with this challenge is for the patient and his circle of caregivers to understand as much as possible about the disease including prognosis, treatment, and potential complications. Moreover, acute leukemia usually demands urgent treatment; the timeframe for absorbing an incredible amount of information is short. Being "completely overwhelmed" or being "hit by a truck" are common phrases used by patients to describe these initial few days after they learn the diagnosis.

The responsibility of the doctor and the patient care team is to inform the patient and his family about the nature of leukemia, the treatment plan, and the implications of the proposed therapy. The transmission of this information is an incredibly difficult process for both the patient and the healthcare team. It takes time, which is a rare commodity in a busy oncology practice. Repetition is also desirable because it is impossible for even the most intellectually gifted person to absorb all this information during a period of great stress. A resource in which the answers to most commonly discussed questions is badly needed as a supplement to what the doctors and nurses can impart.

The monograph by Dr. Ball provides an incredibly useful resource for patients, caregivers, and health care professionals alike. Answers are provided to the most basic questions such as "What is leukemia?" all the way to "What are the functions of a caregiver?" and "What is the responsibility of the patient's employer?" Virtually every question that a patient has asked me over the course of my 30-year career in treating patients with leukemia is answered in a meaningful, straightforward, and easy to understand (without being simplistic) fashion in this text. While monographs provided by groups such as the Leukemia and Lymphoma Society, the MDS Foundation, and the Aplastic Anemia and Myelodysplastic Syndrome Foundation can be very helpful, this treatise is much more thorough. The book represents a resource to which the patient can repeatedly refer during the course of the illness and hopefully post-illness recovery.

What is particularly nice about this text is the breadth of what is covered. Usually I spend a good deal of time discussing bone marrow and blood function as well as the treatment plan and the complications. What receives short shrift are the important questions patients and their families and friends inevitably have about how to be a patient and how to be a caregiver. For example, the chapter on treatment facilities and healthcare providers strikes an extremely good balance between establishing trust in the healthcare team and the importance of the patient and his or her family to be their own advocate.

The treatment of leukemia is becoming an increasingly complex and demanding endeavor. However, success depends on what the patient can understand, tolerate, and expect. The tabulation in *100 Questions & Answers About Leukemia, Third Edition*, provides an extraordinarily useful resource to aid in coping and in making the transitions from diagnosis to treatment to post-treatment to a normal life style and life expectancy.

Richard Stone, MD
Clinical Director, Adult Leukemia Program
Dana Farber Cancer Institute
Associate Professor, Harvard Medical School

Hearing the words, "I am sorry, you have leukemia" in 1997 was the start of the ride of my life. A new way of existence began. A strange (medical) language had to be conquered, making it possible to communicate with those who were treating me. I had to develop completely unknown characteristics for me—patience and trust. Worse, I had to rely on others for survival, a terrible thought at age 45—not to mention dealing with pain, depression, and many months on chemotherapy drugs.

I am here, and I am alive. A wonder to those around me. To get to this point, significant challenges were overcome, not just by me, but by others around me who gave so much of themselves to let me continue to live. No appreciative words can be said that would generate the feelings that I have for all the help and love I was awarded. I am grateful to my fantastic support partners at work, the medical staff from Fred Hutchinson in Seattle and UCSD in San Diego, the continuous prayers from my church members, my donor, and most of all my wife—the greatest caregiver and best friend anyone could have.

Why must we face such challenges? Surely we can do without all this trouble and grief. God apparently thinks not. Romans 5:3-4 says, "…we also rejoice in our sufferings, because we know that suffering produces perseverance; perseverance, character; and character, hope." When we run into problems and trials, we discover that they are good for us—they help us learn to be patient. And patience develops strength of character in us and helps us trust God more each time we use it, until finally our hope and faith are strong and steady.

Finding *the* treatment or regimen that will work against leukemia is the constant challenge for physicians and support staff—a challenge made all the greater by the fact that we are all unique creations, and thus what works for one may not for others. Fine-tuning treatments, learning from experience, and envisioning new ways of healing are the art portion of medical arts and sciences. Although we understand some of the ways that the entire body, mind, and spirit interact in disease and health, there are still many aspects of disease and healing that we don't yet grasp—and there are many great advances that still lie ahead, to be uncovered in the future by the diligent searching—and occasional inspirations—of the people who seek cures for leukemia and other cancers. In the end, though, it is the Master, the One who created us all, who is the true doctor and healer.

Gregory A. Lelek
May 2002

Gregory passed away on June 27, 2006

We have received considerable positive feedback on the first and second editions of *100 Questions & Answers About Leukemia* from patients and colleagues. The diagnosis of leukemia is an overwhelming event for patients and families alike. We have tried to anticipate the questions that inevitably arise when one is faced with this new challenge in life. The *Third Edition* has updated current scientific knowledge. In particular, the treatment of Chronic Myeloid Leukemia (CML) has been revolutionized by the use of a class of drugs called tyrosine kinase inhibitors. The first of these, Gleevec, has become the treatment of choice for CML and has almost completely eliminated allogeneic stem cell transplantation as a treatment for this disease. New drugs in development are adding to this arsenal to fight CML. Progress in the acute leukemias has been slower. The dichotomy in acute leukemia is that we are able to cure a substantial portion of patients with AML but there are still disease-resistant mechanisms that stubbornly refuse to reveal themselves.

The original co-author of this book, Mr. Gregory A. Lelek, was a CML survivor. He underwent an allogeneic stem cell transplant from an unrelated donor many years ago. While it appeared that his CML was cured, he began to experience some respiratory problems and ultimately died of progressive pneumonia. He was a courageous man who fought and won against leukemia, but ultimately succumbed to unrelated causes. I wish to acknowledge his contribution to the original book. I again welcome my new co-author, Mr. Alex Kagan, who also has CML. Alex was a lively contributor to the *Second Edition* and continues to participate in this *Third Edition*.

PART ONE

The Basics

What is leukemia?

What is blood composed of and what
blood cells are affected by leukemia?

How does leukemia affect my immune system?

More . . .

1. What is leukemia?

Leukemia literally means an excess of white blood cells in the blood. Leukemia is a malignant disease (that is, a cancer) of white blood cells in which there are too many white blood cells in the blood and the bone marrow. There are several types of leukemia, but they all have in common the uncontrolled growth of one of the several types of white blood cells. There are four major subtypes of leukemia and several rare forms. The major kinds of leukemia are:

1. Acute myeloid leukemia (AML)
2. Chronic myeloid leukemia (CML)
3. Acute lymphoblastic leukemia (ALL)
4. Chronic lymphocytic leukemia (CLL)

Other, rare types of leukemia include hairy cell leukemia, Sézary cell leukemia, plasma cell leukemia, prolymphocytic leukemia, and the leukemic phase of lymphoma.

Leukemia is a serious and life-threatening disease. It might seem odd that having too many white blood cells is dangerous because white blood cells fight disease. So how can you have too much of a good thing? As described later, cancerous white blood cells do not behave the way normal white blood cells do, so they cannot fight disease effectively. If the bone marrow (see Question 5) overproduces these cancerous cells at the expense of normal cells, the leukemia patient can soon end up with insufficient numbers of the normal cells to fight off the daily challenge of infections. Furthermore, the overproduction of abnormal white blood cells leads to decreased production of other important blood cells, including red blood cells and platelets. For this reason, leukemia is a very serious, potentially fatal condition.

2. What is blood composed of and what blood cells are affected by leukemia?

As you know, blood is a red liquid that is vital to life. Blood is composed of water as well as a multitude of different proteins,

Figure 1

including antibodies and important hormones and transport molecules; nutritional products, such as sugars, fats, and amino acids; and most importantly for the topic of this book, living cells. The major types of blood cells are **leukocytes** (also known as **white blood cells**), **red blood cells** (cells that contain hemoglobin and carry oxygen to the tissues), and **platelets** (cells necessary for blood clotting and formed in the blood marrow) (see **Figure 1**). All blood cells are manufactured in the bone marrow, growing from a cell known as the hematopoietic stem cell (see Question 32). Leukemia is a malignancy (cancer) of the white blood cell. However, there are several types of white blood cells (**Figure 2**).

Lymphocytes are one type of white blood cell that can be further broken down into **B lymphocytes** and **T lymphocytes**. B lymphocytes, which are the minority, make antibody molecules, which are secreted by these cells and can then attach to substances called **antigens**. An antigen can either be a soluble molecule (a protein dissolved in liquid blood) or possibly a protein attached to or part of a foreign cell such as a bacterium, fungus, or cancer cell (a cell that divides

Leukocyte

A white blood cell or corpuscle.

White blood cells

Blood cells that do not contain hemoglobin; also called leukocytes.

Red blood cells

Hemoglobin-containing cells that carry oxygen to the tissues.

Lymphocytes

Weakly mobile cells made in lymphoid tissue that are typical cellular elements of lymph and include cellular mediators of immunity; constitute 20%–30% of leukocytes of normal human blood.

Summary of Blood Cells

Name	Light Micrograph	Description	Concentration (Number of Cells/mm³)	Life Span	Function
Red blood cells (RBCs)		Biconcave disk; no nucleus	4–6 million	120 days	Transports oxygen and carbon dioxide
White blood cells Neutrophil		Approximately twice the size of RBCs; multi-lobed nucleus; clear-staining cytoplasm	3000 to 7000	6 hours to a few days	Phagocytizes bacteria
Eosinophil		Approximately same size as neutrophil; large pink-staining granules; bilobed nucleus	100 to 400	8–12 days	Phagocytizes antigen-antibody complex; attacks parasites
Basophil		Slightly smaller than neutrophil; contains large, purple cytoplasmic granules; bilobed nucleus	20 to 50	Few hours to a few days	Releases histamine during inflammation
Monocyte		Larger than neutrophil; cytoplasm grayish-blue; no cytoplasmic granules; U- or kidney-shaped nucleus	100 to 700	Lasts many months	Phagocytizes bacteria, dead cells, and cellular debris
Lymphocyte		Slightly smaller than neutrophil; large, relatively round nucleus that fills the cell	1500 to 3000	Can persist many years	Involved in immune protection, either attacking cells directly or producing antibodies
Platelets		Fragments of megakaryocytes; appear as small dark-staining granules	250,000	5–10 days	Play several key roles in blood clotting

Figure 2

B lymphocytes

Subset of lymphocytes that makes antibodies.

T lymphocytes

Subset of lymphocytes that directly attach themselves to virally infected or transformed cells to mediate their destruction.

and reproduces abnormally with uncontrolled growth). T lymphocytes directly attach themselves to cells infected or transformed by viruses to help destroy them.

Another type of white blood cell is the **monocyte**, or, once it is specialized (differentiated) in tissues, the **macrophage**.

The monocyte is important for a couple of reasons. The first is that monocytes are highly effective at digesting foreign antigens, such as those from an invading virus, and presenting them to T lymphocytes to generate an immune response in order to protect the individual. This is the primary way that long-term immunity against invading microorganisms works. The second function of monocytes is that they are able to ingest, or engulf, invading **microorganisms** (organisms of minute, microscopic size) or cells that have been targeted by **antibodies**.

The third type of white blood cell is the granulocyte, a term that refers to the large numbers of granules in these cells. The most common granulocyte is a cell called the neutrophil. The neutrophil is highly effective at recognizing and killing bacteria and other microorganisms. The absence of neutrophils is perhaps the worst consequence of acute leukemia because the body's ability to fight off bacterial and fungal conditions is virtually nonexistent when the body is empty of neutrophils.

All blood cells arise from a class of cells called stem cells (see Question 32). The bone marrow stem cell is called the hematopoietic stem cell, referring to its ability to make all the cellular elements of the blood. The stem cell is capable of renewing itself during cell division, but it is also capable of undergoing a process called **differentiation**. At the start of this process, the stem cell goes through several stages of development, which result in more specialized stem cells with limited differentiation capabilities, which finally give rise to each of the various blood elements. Leukemia appears to be initiated by genetic events (i.e., inherited patterns for certain characteristics) occurring in the stem cell at a particular stage in development. Thus, the type of leukemia that arises has something to do with the exact nature of the genetic event and the cell in which the event occurs. If the malignant transformation occurs in a neutrophil precursor, the disease **acute myeloid leukemia** (AML) arises. If the disease is begun by a particular molecular event in the stem cell, a disease known as **chronic myeloid leukemia** (CML) develops. If the disease is initiated in a stem cell that has differentiated into the lymphoid lineage, the resulting leukemia will be a lymphocytic leukemia of either B cells or T cells, known as **acute lymphocytic leukemia** (ALL). Finally, a particular subset of lymphocytes appears to be susceptible

Antigen

Substance capable of stimulating an immune response.

Monocyte

A type of white blood cell that is transported to tissues, where it turns into a macrophage.

The absence of neutrophils is perhaps the worst consequence of acute leukemia because the body's ability to fight off bacterial and fungal conditions is virtually nonexistent when the body is empty of neutrophils.

The Basics

5

Macrophage

A cell derived from a monocyte that functions to protect against infection and noxious substances.

Microorganism

An organism of minute, microscopic size.

Antibody

Any of the body's immunoglobulins that are produced in response to specific antigens.

Differentiation

The process during which the stem cell goes through several stages of development.

Acute myeloid leukemia

Rapidly growing leukemia affecting mature white cells.

Chronic myeloid leukemia

A slow-growing leukemia of mature white blood cells, associated with the Philadelphia chromosome.

Acute lymphocytic leukemia

Rapidly growing leukemia affecting lymphocytes.

to malignancy, giving rise to the disease **chronic lymphocytic leukemia** (CLL).

3. How does leukemia affect my immune system?

Leukemia depresses your **immune system** (a complex system by which the body protects itself from outside invaders that are harmful to it) somewhat indirectly. On one hand, the presence of the large numbers of leukemia cells crowds out the normal cells of the immune system, which causes **immunosuppression** (i.e., lowered resistance to disease). In addition, the treatment of leukemia can further depress the number of normal immune system cells and further contribute to immunosuppression. In general, the immunosuppression is specific for fairly common microorganisms, such as bacteria and fungi that are all around us naturally. When the levels of normal white blood cells that ordinarily keep us from getting infected are decreased, these common bugs can become quite aggressive and can enter the blood and tissues.

4. What are risk factors for leukemia?

Leukemia seems to arise from damage or alterations occurring in the DNA that, in turn, affect various genes. Thus, DNA-damaging agents are known initiators of leukemia. These include certain chemicals, such as benzene and other solvents; ionizing radiation; and some other organic compounds, including, paradoxically, chemotherapy drugs, that is, drugs used to treat other cancers. In fact, so-called **secondary leukemia** (i.e., leukemia caused by chemotherapy) is fairly common in patients previously treated with certain types of chemotherapy for breast cancer, Hodgkin's disease, and multiple myeloma. The incidence of secondary AML approaches 5% in certain subgroups of patients treated in this manner. Obviously, this is a great tragedy, and efforts to modify chemotherapy regimens to reduce the incidence of secondary leukemia are ongoing. Leukemia is also age dependent. Children are at higher risk for

ALL, and adults are more at risk for CLL. Adults are increasingly at risk for AML as they age; the incidence of this disease increases even more rapidly in patients over the age of 60 years. CML begins to occur in young adults to middle-aged adults, but it is slightly less common in older adults. Certain **congenital diseases** are associated with a higher incidence of leukemia, including Down syndrome, Bloom syndrome, and ataxia telangiectasia. Leukemia also occurs in twice as many patients who smoke cigarettes compared with those who do not.

Do electrical power lines cause leukemia? This issue has been raised numerous times in the past. Many studies have been conducted, but none has found any evidence to support the theory that living near power lines can cause leukemia. There are occasional reports of clusters of cases of leukemia in a community. These sorts of events raise the question of whether some local exposure to toxins or poisons, radioactivity, or electrical power lines is the culprit. However, studies are usually inconclusive, and often, no good explanation for the clustering is ever discovered.

In fact, in most patients with leukemia, the disease does not have any identifiable cause. That is, most patients have not worked in occupations that exposed them to toxic substances, they have not taken known leukemia-inciting drugs, and they have not been exposed to radiation above the usual levels that an average person would be exposed to in the course of life, such as from dental X-ray studies or an occasional chest X-ray study. It seems that an accident occurs during cell division in the bone marrow in which a mutation occurs in the genome that suddenly triggers the onset of the disease. Perhaps it is related to the extraordinarily high rate of cell division that takes place every day in the bone marrow and the blood, leading to the inevitability that occasionally accidents will occur during the process of duplicating the DNA during cell division.

Chronic lymphocytic leukemia

A slow-growing leukemia that affects mature lymphocytes.

Immune system

Complex system by which the body protects itself from outside invaders that are harmful to it.

Immunosuppression

Condition of having a lowered resistance to disease. May be a temporary result of lowered white blood cells from chemotherapy administration.

Secondary leukemia

A malignancy somewhat more common in patients previously treated with certain types of chemotherapy.

Congenital disease

A disease existing at or dating from birth.

The Basics

5. What is bone marrow?

Bone marrow

The soft, fatty substance filling the cavities of the bones. Blood cells are made here.

Bone marrow is a soft, fatty substance inside bones where all of the blood cells are made. Some of the bone marrow is so-called red bone marrow, which is where the blood cells are made. Some is so-called yellow bone marrow, which is largely replaced by fat. The red bone marrow is predominantly found in the skull, vertebral bodies, ribs, sternum, and pelvis. There is a complicated architecture inside the bone, where the bone marrow cells reside. Although the bone marrow cavity is separated from the blood circulation by a membrane, they are still in direct contact with each other. As blood cells are made in the bone marrow cavity, they gradually acquire the ability to mobilize from the marrow into the blood, which is percolating through the bone. Thus, the bone marrow is the site of blood cell production. All blood cells, including lymphocytes, originate from a stem cell (see Question 32) that resides in the bone marrow.

PART TWO

Facts About Leukemia: Risks, Diagnosis, and Effects

Are there different types of leukemia? Why is one called acute and one called chronic?

What is myelodysplastic syndrome? Is it related to leukemia?

What is a blast?

More . . .

6. Are there different types of leukemia? Why is one called acute and one called chronic?

The four major types of leukemia are acute lymphocytic leukemia (ALL), acute myeloid leukemia (AML), chronic lymphocytic leukemia (CLL), and chronic myeloid leukemia (CML). The term **acute** is applied to leukemias that present abruptly and are characterized by large numbers of very immature, undifferentiated cells that, if untreated, rapidly lead to the death of the patient. The term **chronic** applies to leukemias that grow more slowly and less dramatically, thus leading to a much longer life span for the afflicted individual, even without treatment.

Acute Lymphoblastic Leukemia

ALL is a cancer of lymphocytes that often begins in a rapid, dramatic manner. ALL is the most common cancer in children, but it also occurs in adults. There are three different subtypes of ALL, based on the appearance of the leukemic, or blast (imperfectly developing) cells. These subtypes are termed *L1* (most common in children), *L2* (most common in adults), and *L3*, the most aggressive, also called Burkitt-like leukemia. The treatment of ALL is complicated. Multiple chemotherapeutic drugs are used in a phase called **induction chemotherapy** to induce a **remission** (a complete or partial disappearance of the signs and symptoms of the cancer) (see Table 1 and Questions 23 and 24). After this, **intensification chemotherapy** using more chemotherapy drugs is required to achieve the desired goal of a cure. This phase of therapy is designed to eliminate any leukemia cells that were missed by induction chemotherapy. In addition, the spinal fluid often is invaded by ALL cells, leading to the need to either treat or prevent spinal fluid involvement with ALL, using drugs introduced into the spinal fluid through a lumbar puncture or through a device inserted into the brain called an **Ommaya reservoir**. After a remission is achieved, patients with ALL must continue to undergo treatment for a full 2 years.

Table 1 Medications Commonly Used for Treating Different Leukemias

Type of Leukemia	Generic Name	Trade Name
AML	Cytarabine*	Cytosar-U
	Daunorubicin	Cerubidine
	Gemtuzumab ozogamicin	Mylotarg
	Idarubicin	Idamycin
	Mitoxantrone	Novantrone
	VP–16	Etoposide
ALL	6-mercaptopurine	Purinethol
	6-thioguanine	Tabloid
	L-asparaginase	Oncaspar Elspar Erwinaze
	Clofarabine	
	Cyclophosphamide	Cytoxan
	Cytarabine*	Cytosar-U
	Daunorubicin	Cerubidine
	Methotrexate, amethopterin	Folex
	Nelarabine	Arranon
	Prednisone	Deltasone
	Vincristine	Oncovin
CML	Dasatinib	Sprycel
	Hydroxyurea	Hydrea
	Imatinib mesylate	Gleevec, Glivec
	Interferon alpha	Intron A
	Nilotinib	Tasigna
CLL	Alemtuzumab	Campath
	Bendamustine	Treanda
	Chlorambucil	Leukeran
	Cyclophosphamide	Cytoxan
	Fludarabine	Fludara
	Ofatumumab	Arzerra
	Prednisone	Deltasone
	Rituximab	Rituxan

* Cytarabine is also called ara-c.

Facts About Leukemia: Risks, Diagnosis, and Effects

The cure rate of childhood ALL is very high, approaching 75% of patients.

Bone marrow transplant

A procedure in which the bone marrow of a leukemia patient is replaced by another person's marrow.

Complete remission

Total absence of disease.

Consolidation

Additional chemotherapy after remission, often given in cycles.

The cure rate of childhood ALL is very high, approaching 75% of patients. The cure rate in adult ALL patients is not quite as good, but it has improved steadily over the years. One subgroup of patients with ALL has previously been considered to have a worse prognosis: those having the Philadelphia chromosome in the leukemia cells. These patients are still usually referred for a **bone marrow transplant**, described in Part 4. New medications that target the genetic cause of this subtype of ALL, such as imatinib mesylate (Gleevec) or dasatinib (Sprycel), are now included in the treatment regimens for Philadelphia chromosome-positive ALL. In the absence of the Philadelphia chromosome, the cure rate for adult ALL is approximately 40% with chemotherapy alone, and there is increasing evidence that bone marrow transplantation following induction chemotherapy improves upon the results of chemotherapy in adult patients (see Questions 32–42).

Acute Myeloid Leukemia

AML usually affects adults. The incidence increases with age, and many patients develop AML as a consequence of treatment for other cancers. This disease usually has a very rapid onset, with obvious symptoms such as fatigue, fever, infection, and bleeding. Untreated, it is rapidly fatal. However, treatment with chemotherapy is highly effective at achieving **complete remission** (see Questions 21 and 22). Therapy must be initiated as soon as possible in a hospital setting. Complete remissions (total absence of disease) are obtained in 50% to 80% of patients, with older patients having less favorable results than younger patients. There are eight subtypes of AML, as defined by the French American British (FAB) system, labeled M0 through M7. One of the subtypes, M3, is treated with chemotherapy and a differentiating agent called all-trans-retinoic acid (ATRA) (see Question 23). The other six subtypes are treated in a fairly consistent manner. Induction chemotherapy (i.e., initial chemotherapy), usually consisting of cytosine arabinoside and one other drug, is used to induce a remission. After remission is achieved, **consolidation** (i.e., repeated cycles of chemotherapy) must be pursued, or almost all patients will **relapse** (i.e., experience a reappearance of cancer after a disease-free period). Consolidation can consist of more chemotherapy, given in cycles, usually at least twice at approximately monthly intervals. Consolidation might also include **autologous** (using cells from the patient's own body) or **allogeneic stem cell transplantation** (using cells from another's body) (see Questions 35 and 36). The overall cure rate for all patients with AML is only about 25%. However, certain subgroups fare much better, depending on the patient's age, the prognostic factors, and the exact treatment that the patient receives.

Chronic Myeloid Leukemia

CML is a disease that occurs primarily in adults. It is manifested by a high white blood cell count and sometimes by a high platelet count. The disease is often diagnosed by chance because it is a chronic, slow-growing process that does not produce any symptoms before the white count starts to rise. CML usually evolves into a more aggressive phase first, called accelerated phase, and then a worse phase called **blastic crisis**. Blastic crisis refers to the tendency of CML cells to lose their ability to differentiate into mature white blood cells. At this phase of the disease, the cells behave very much like cells in AML—they grow rapidly, replacing the normal bone marrow cells, thus leading to low platelets and red blood cells. This phase of CML requires treatment similar to AML, but it actually has a worse prognosis than AML. Once the acute phase has occurred, if a remission is achieved with chemotherapy (including the new drug imatinib mesylate, discussed later), a bone marrow transplant should be strongly considered.

The treatment of CML has undergone a revolution. Previously, patients could be treated with an oral drug, hydroxyurea, for a short time to decrease the white blood cell count, or they might receive interferon alpha. Bone marrow transplantation was frequently used in the first, chronic phase of their disease to attempt to cure it, and in fact, transplantation is considered the only known curative therapy for this disease (see Questions

Relapse

The reappearance of cancer after a disease-free period.

Autologous

Coming from the same person.

Allogeneic stem cell transplantation

Cells from another's body are used to treat a cancer.

Blast crisis

The evolution of CML in the chronic phase to an acute and aggressive leukemia much like AML.

32–42). Imatinib mesylate (Gleevec) (see Question 22) was approved in 2001 for use with CML by the United States **Food and Drug Administration** (FDA), the federal agency responsible for approving and regulating medications, foods, and other products for human consumption. This oral drug, which is relatively free of side effects, produces sustained remissions in a high proportion of patients with this disease. In a small percentage of patients, resistance to imatinib mesylate develops through a mutation in the abnormal protein that imatinib mesylate targets. Another oral drug that inhibits the same protein as imatinib mesylate, but is not affected by the mutations in the same manner, has also recently been approved by the FDA. This drug, dasatinib (Sprycel), targets two proteins in CML cells and can be additive to the effects of imatinib mesylate. Patients who have incomplete responses to imatinib mesylate or who are intolerant due to side effects now may be treated with dasatinib. Yet another tyrosine kinase inhibitor, nilotinib (Tasigna), was also approved for CML. The best choice of agent to treat CML is still under study. The good news for patients is that they have a choice of three different medications that work very well and are very safe, though not without some side effects.

As mentioned previously, the natural history of CML is that the relative slow progress of the disease gives way to a more acute form of the disease—the blastic phase that is similar to AML. The current question with imatinib mesylate is how long will it prevent the onset of a blast crisis? Recent follow-up data from the original clinical trial of imatinib mesylate that led to its FDA approval are very encouraging. Many patients have been on treatment with imatinib for over 10 years with no signs of progression to blast crisis.

The need for bone marrow transplantation is less frequent now because of the use and efficacy of new oral drugs such as imatinib mesylate. Patients are generally not recommended for transplantation unless their disease becomes resistant to the tyrosine kinases. However, if and when the disease process

Food and Drug Administration

A federal institution charged with approving and regulating medications, foodstuff, and other products for human consumption.

accelerates, or if resistance to imatinib mesylate and the other agents develops, allogeneic bone marrow transplant is still the only known curative therapy for CML.

Chronic Lymphocytic Leukemia

CLL is a disease that exclusively affects adults. It is unusual for patients to be diagnosed with CLL under the age of 40, and most patients who are diagnosed are over the age of 60. This is a slowly progressing disease in which the lymphocytes gradually increase in the blood, and eventually in the lymph nodes and spleen. The natural history is a very slow but progressive accumulation of these abnormal yet innocuous lymphocytes. As in other leukemias, the problem arises when the normal blood cells are sufficiently suppressed by the proliferating lymphocytes. Treatment of CLL is also undergoing an evolution because of the introduction of new drugs. Some patients are being treated with oral chemotherapy agents, but increasingly intravenous agents such as fludarabine (Fludara), cyclophosphamide (Cytoxan), and a recently approved drug called bendamustine (Treanda) are employed (see Questions 23 and 24). Biologic therapy, including monoclonal antibodies and gene therapy (still experimental), is increasingly used in the treatment of CLL (see Question 27). Some patients undergo bone marrow transplantation, which can be curative in CLL. Patients with fludarabine-resistant disease or those who have particularly poor prognostic markers for disease progression are the ideal candidates for stem cell transplantation. Transplantation is limited to relatively young patients with suitably matched donors (see Questions 32–42).

7. What is myelodysplastic syndrome? Is it related to leukemia?

Myelodysplastic syndrome (MDS) is a disease of the bone marrow stem cells in which the normal maturation of blood cells is altered. The cause is unknown, but exposure to chemicals, solvent, and toxins are responsible for some cases. The syndrome is recognized by the finding of low blood counts; usually two or more of the major blood cell elements are present in low levels in the blood. As the disorder progresses, blood transfusions might become necessary. MDS often leads to acute myeloid leukemia (AML). Roughly one third of MDS patients will eventually have AML. The other two thirds will eventually succumb to complications relating to their low blood counts, such as infection and uncontrolled bleeding.

Supportive treatment

Treatment with the goal of preserving the strength of the patient.

Hematopoietic growth factors

Drugs that increase blood cell counts.

Treatment of MDS is generally **supportive** (i.e., with the goal of preserving the strength of the patient) because there is no proven treatment that directly treats the underlying disease. **Hematopoietic growth factors**, such as granulocyte colony-stimulating factor (G-CSF, filgrastim; see Question 43) and erythropoietin (Procrit or Aranesp), might help some patients by elevating the blood counts. Drugs such as thalidomide and lenalidomide (Revlimid) are currently undergoing clinical trials to determine their ability to help patients with MDS (see Question 29). Lenalidomide is approved by the FDA for the treatment of one of the types of MDS that is associated with deletions of part of chromosome 5 called 5q-minus syndrome. Other therapies that have recently been approved include the agents 5-azacytidine (Vidaza) and decitabine (Dacogen). These agents are believed to work by unblocking the ability of the MDS cells to differentiate and thus make healthy blood cells. Both are increasingly used to treat MDS patients with some success in a substantial proportion of patients.

Diagnosis

The process of identifying a disease by its characteristic signs, symptoms, and laboratory findings.

Prognosis

A prediction of the course of the disease; the future prospect for the patient.

Cytopenia

Low blood count.

At the time of **diagnosis** (the process of identifying a disease by its characteristic signs, symptoms, and laboratory results), a doctor estimates the future course of the disease (i.e., the **prognosis**) and potential for the patient's survival by considering certain features of the disease. These include the percentage of blasts in the bone marrow, the existence of certain cytogenetic abnormalities (see Question 18), and the number of **cytopenias** (low blood counts, either red blood cells, white blood cells, or platelets).

Patients with advanced MDS might be treated as if they have leukemia (because they almost have leukemia anyway). This treatment might restore relatively normal bone marrow function, similar to a remission in leukemia. Patients with high-risk MDS or whose disease has progressed to leukemia, and who have a histocompatibility antigen (HLA)-matched sibling or an unrelated donor should strongly consider an **allogeneic bone marrow transplantation** (bone marrow transplantation using marrow from another person's body) rather than chemotherapy. This procedure is curative in about 50% of cases.

8. *What is a blast?*

A **blast** is an immature white blood cell that normally represents an early phase of the normal differentiation process that occurs in the bone marrow. Patients with AML or ALL have excess numbers of these cells in the bone marrow and usually the blood as well. In fact, it is the presence of large numbers of these cells that allows the diagnosis of leukemia. The goal of treatment of the leukemia is to decrease the numbers of these cells to normal levels (*normal* means that fewer than 5% of the bone marrow cells are blasts). Sometimes, it is difficult to tell the difference between normal and malignant blasts when the number of blasts is low. More specific tests, such as flow cytometry and cytogenetic analysis (see Question 18), are then used to help distinguish normal from leukemia-related blasts. A doctor will monitor the levels of blast cells in a patient's blood and bone marrow to assess the status of leukemia and its response to therapy. It is almost always abnormal to have blasts in the blood. Therefore, the doctor will monitor blood counts (tests to measure the number of red blood cells, white blood cells, and platelets in blood) and look for any blasts periodically during the treatment of the leukemia and afterward to ensure that the disease is still in remission.

Allogeneic bone marrow transplantation

Bone marrow transplantation using marrow from another person's body.

Blast

An immature white blood cell that normally represents an early phase of the normal differentiation process that occurs in the bone marrow.

9. What is a platelet?

A **platelet** is a tiny cell that is found in the blood. It is responsible for plugging up small holes that might develop in the blood vessels, and therefore, it is the first defense against bleeding. Platelets originally come from a cell in the bone marrow called a megakaryocyte. Patients with acute leukemia commonly have low platelet counts; low platelet counts carry a higher risk for spontaneous bleeding (bleeding with no obvious cause). Therefore, the number of platelets is monitored, and if it is particularly low, platelet transfusions (see Question 50) might be given to keep the platelet level to a suitable level. Patients with CML can actually have high platelet counts when the disease is first diagnosed. Despite this, sometimes the platelets don't work as well as they should, so bleeding can occur in CML as well. The platelet count in patients with CLL is normal in the early stages. In later stages, it is often low, either because of decreased production of platelets in the bone marrow or because of increased destruction of platelets from an **autoimmune process** (i.e., when a person's immune system reacts against tissues in his or her own body). This autoimmune process might be treated with **immunosuppressive therapy** (i.e., therapy to decrease the response of the immune system; this treatment is intended to treat the autoimmune process), including prednisone, intravenous immunoglobulin, and splenectomy (removal of the spleen).

10. How common is leukemia?

Leukemia is a relatively uncommon form of cancer. Currently, leukemia represents about 3% of all cancer in the United States and has an annual **incidence** (the number of new cases of leukemia occurring during a certain period) of about 37,000. The acute leukemias and the chronic leukemias occur with about the same frequency. However, because patients with CML and CLL on average live longer than those with AML and ALL, the **prevalence** (the number of people alive at any moment) of chronic leukemia is greater.

Table 2   Expected Incidence of Leukemia in 2010

Type of Leukemia	Age*	Incidence
AML	65 years	12,330
CML	50 years	4870
ALL	2–3 years, 65 years	5330
CLL	55 years	14,990

* Indicates median age, that is, the number at the exact midpoint of the spectrum. Half the cases are below and half are above the median age.

Children are more likely to develop ALL than any other form of cancer in general. AML is the second most common leukemia in children, but is much less common than ALL. Although a rare form of juvenile CML occurs in infants and very young children, CML and CLL do not commonly occur in children.

Young adults are more likely to get AML or CML than ALL or CLL. It is very unusual for someone to contract CLL before the age of 40. However, CLL then becomes increasingly common with advancing age, as do all of the leukemias. In fact, the incidence of AML and ALL increases sharply after the age of 60 years. Therefore, as the population continues to live longer, it is expected that leukemia will be diagnosed more often in the upcoming decades. Table 2 illustrates the expected incidence of each type of leukemia in the year 2010 in the United States, as projected by the Leukemia and Lymphoma Society.

11. Is leukemia inherited? Does it run in families?

The vast majority of patients with leukemia have no family history of leukemia. Furthermore, there is no evidence that leukemia can be passed on to the children of a person with leukemia. That said, there are occasional families with two or more members who have developed leukemia or related illnesses. This phenomenon suggests that there might be a genetic predisposition to develop leukemia, analogous to the known increased susceptibility that some people have to develop certain other forms of cancer, such as breast cancer. However, at this time, the genetic or molecular basis for leukemia susceptibility is unknown. People with certain genetic diseases such as Down syndrome, Bloom syndrome, and ataxia telangiectasia are more susceptible to leukemia for as-yet unknown reasons (see Question 4).

Leukemia occasionally occurs in pregnant women, and most commonly, it is either AML or CML, because the childbearing age coincides with the usual age of onset of these diseases. Obviously, the diagnosis of leukemia in a pregnant woman presents a very serious medical problem and is an emotional tragedy for the parents. What to do regarding therapy depends on the stage of the pregnancy in which the illness is diagnosed. If the diagnosis is made during the first trimester, termination of the pregnancy might be considered because the woman cannot usually wait more than 6 months to begin therapy. Chemotherapeutic drugs are known mutagens and **carcinogens** (substances that initiate or promote the development of cancer). Thus, they should not be used in the early phases of pregnancy. A woman in the second or third trimester might be treated supportively (i.e., to maintain her strength) until childbirth if the disease is not too aggressive. However, if she has AML, she might need to be treated with chemotherapy before delivery. This has been done many times with no clear detriment to the child. On the other hand, waiting to treat until delivery places the mother at greater risk of dying from the leukemia.

Carcinogen

Any substance that initiates or promotes the development of cancer.

12. Is leukemia contagious? Can leukemia be acquired through a blood transfusion?

No. The only exception to this is the rare virus HTLV–1, which can cause a rare form of T-cell disease with some features of leukemia. It is found in certain areas, such as the

Caribbean and Japan, and it is transmitted by sexual and bodily fluid contact. However, for the common forms of leukemia, there should be no fear that contact with others could spread the illness.

Some people have wondered if an animal disease, such as feline leukemia, causes leukemia in humans. Many viruses cause cancer, including leukemia, in animals. However, these viruses have never been found to be present in any humans with leukemia. There is absolutely no evidence of transmission of leukemia to a human being from an animal.

In a **blood transfusion**, the red blood cells are replaced in the bloodstream when a person's own bone marrow is unable to replace them. Because there is no known external cause of leukemia, such as a virus, the only way leukemia could be acquired through a blood transfusion would be by the direct introduction of leukemia cells into the recipient. However, because the cells of a random blood donor would be detected as foreign by the recipient, they would be destroyed immediately. There is simply no evidence that leukemia has ever been acquired from a blood transfusion.

Blood transfusion

Replenishment of red blood cells in the bloodstream when one's own bone marrow is unable to do so.

There is simply no evidence that leukemia has ever been acquired from a blood transfusion.

13. Does diet play a role in my getting ill?

There is no evidence that any dietary exposure or deficiency can influence the onset of leukemia or its behavior once it is diagnosed. A balanced diet, meaning a diet containing the recommended proportions of the various food groups (vegetables, grains, dairy products, and meat) and vitamins, is certainly recommended for you (as it is for anyone!). This is because a healthy body will help you tolerate the treatment you will need for your leukemia. But caution is advised for the use of any special diets in the hopes of improving the likelihood of cure. There is no credible evidence that eating a special diet will cure your disease. Dietary supplements should be avoided unless your doctor specifically advises you that it is safe to take them. The FDA does not regulate or approve of most supplements, allowing unsubstantiated, often erroneous claims to go unchallenged (see Question 54). If you are neutropenic, meaning that your body is depleted of important disease-fighting white blood cells, you will be told to avoid certain fresh fruits and vegetables because they can harbor dangerous microorganisms that could cause illness (see Question 15).

Of course, a discussion of a healthy lifestyle must mention issues such as cigarette smoking, alcohol use, and exercise. Smoking cigarettes will not help you in your fight with leukemia. For one thing, your lungs will be more susceptible to infection. For another, your heart can be adversely affected if it has to work harder to pump blood because of the effects on your lungs. Alcohol use needs to be avoided or restricted to very small quantities, and you should particularly avoid it when you're in an especially vulnerable condition, such as when you are experiencing low platelets or white blood cells. Alcohol affects the ability of the marrow to regenerate and also depresses the function of normal white blood cells and platelets. If you are already a smoker and find that you suddenly need to be treated for leukemia, nicotine patches can be used to decrease the side effects of sudden smoking cessation.

There is no evidence that any nutritional factor causes leukemia, but cigarette smoking has been found to increase the incidence of AML by twofold. An excellent article summarizing the roles of nutrition and physical activity in cancer prevention can be found at the American Cancer Society's web site at *www.cancer.org*.

14. How does someone know he or she has leukemia?

Leukemia can become evident in many different ways. In fact, some patients have no symptoms at all, and the only reason the disease is diagnosed is because of routine blood testing. For example, at a routine physical, a blood test called a complete blood count (CBC) might be performed (see Question 16), and it might indicate that the white count is high or possibly even low. Alternatively, the platelet count might be depressed, as is common in acute leukemias. Finally, there can be signs of anemia in the CBC, which also could lead to a further examination of the bone marrow.

Many patients, however, do have symptoms that eventually bring them to a physician. Unfortunately, the symptoms are relatively vague. For example, generalized fatigue is very common because of the anemia that many patients experience with leukemia. Infection that is not very responsive to antibiotics or that simply persists for a longer than usual period of time is also a sign of leukemia. Abnormal bleeding might also be noticed. For instance, there might be bleeding in the gums from a low platelet count, or there might be diffuse swelling of the gums in addition to bleeding, which is common in acute myelomonocytic leukemia, one of the common types of AML. Small red dots might appear on the lower parts of the legs or in the oral cavity; these little dots are known as **petechiae** and are due to a very low platelet count. Excessive bruising might be noticed, also due to a low platelet count. Some patients experience a feeling of fullness in their abdomen, especially after eating, due to an enlarged spleen. This is particularly common in CML. Children sometimes experience swollen lymph nodes and perhaps sore joints in association with ALL.

Petechiae

Small red dots on the skin as a result of very low platelet count.

The best general advice is to seek medical attention if you have severe fatigue, abnormal bleeding, or infections that persist. A full examination, including blood work, can usually disclose whether leukemia is present. A final diagnosis is usually made after a bone marrow biopsy and aspiration (see Question 17) are performed. Remember that the overwhelming majority of people who have the symptoms of fatigue and a persistent infection do not have leukemia. However, it is such a serious disease to go undiagnosed that it needs to be considered early in the differential diagnosis of these general complaints.

When a patient is suspected of having leukemia based on his or her symptoms and the results of some initial blood tests, a careful physical examination and a more complete panel of blood tests will be performed, as will a bone marrow aspiration and biopsy. Samples of bone marrow (and possibly the blood as well) will be studied by **flow cytometry** (a test of cancerous tissues that shows the aggressiveness of a **tumor**, which is an abnormal tissue, swelling, or mass) and cytogenetic analysis (see Question 18), and the microscopic appearance of the leukemia cells, if any, will be examined. The results received from all of this testing can take days to weeks to accumulate. At that point, the precise diagnosis of the type and the subtype of leukemia can be made. This leads to the next step, which is treatment. This will all be explained more fully in subsequent questions.

15. What is neutropenia?

Neutropenia refers to a very low level of one of the important white blood cells, the neutrophil. The neutrophil, also known as the polymorphonuclear leukocyte, is a specialized type of white blood cell that protects us from bacterial and fungal pathogens (agents that cause infection). The neutrophil is able to engulf (phagocytose) bacteria that may or may not be coated with antibodies. This protective function is extremely effective at allowing a person to be free of infections caused by bacteria or fungi that are widespread in the environment. For example, bacteria, some of which could cause disease, heavily colonize the mouth and gastrointestinal tract. If defenses are down, they can enter into the bloodstream and cause serious, life-threatening infection. Normally, the neutrophil is situated in the tissues or in the bloodstream in a way that enables it to be the first line of defense against such invasion.

Severe neutropenia is a concentration of neutrophils in the blood of less than 500 cells per cubic millimeter (mm^3) of blood, which is about 20% of normal levels. Generally, there are approximately 2500 neutrophils per mm^3 of blood. When the neutrophil count is less than 500 per mm^3, the rate of bacterial

Flow cytometry

A test performed on cancerous tissues that shows the aggressiveness of the tumor.

Tumor

An abnormal tissue, swelling, or mass; may be either benign or malignant.

Neutropenia

A condition in which the body is depleted of important disease-fighting white blood cells.

and fungal infections is dramatically higher than when the count is above that number. Because the leukemia itself and the chemotherapy used to treat the leukemia are frequently associated with low neutrophil counts, neutropenia is common in patients with leukemia. Therefore, special consideration needs to be given for the patient's protection. A **neutropenic diet** (one that is low in microbes, which might transmit infectious agents, such as bacteria, fungi, or parasites) is important because the ingestion of microscopic amounts of bacteria can result in a serious infection in a patient with a low white blood cell count and/or one who is undergoing treatment with immunosuppressive medications. These microorganisms ordinarily would be contained by the neutrophils, but when neutrophil levels are low, this function is lost, leading to potentially deadly infections. It has recently been recognized that relaxation of certain restrictions is permissible. Your doctor and his/her team will give you the guidelines used at their institution. Secondly, a patient might be treated **prophylactically** with antibiotics to prevent disease or infection. Although the use of prophylactic antibiotics might promote the generation of resistant strains of bacteria or fungi, most physicians would still recommend prophylactic antibiotics for the neutropenic patient because of the high risk of life-threatening infections.

Neutropenic diet

A diet that avoids foods that might carry harmful bacteria, such as raw meats or fresh fruits and vegetables.

Prophylactic treatment

Treatment geared to prevent disease or infection.

16. What is a CBC?

Those who have leukemia will frequently have a blood test called a **complete blood count** (CBC). This is the most important blood test for monitoring leukemia and its response to treatment. A CBC provides the very useful and vital information concerning the levels of the three major blood cells, the red blood cells, the white blood cells, and the platelets (see Questions 1 and 9). Patients may see the results of their blood tests on a laboratory report, which can be confusing because a fairly large number of results are reported, giving one the impression that each is an individual test. In reality, the important numbers are the WBC (white blood count), the hct (the hematocrit, meaning the percentage of red blood

Complete blood count

A laboratory test to determine the number of red blood cells, white blood cells, platelets, hemoglobin, and other components of a blood sample.

cells in the blood), the hgb (the concentration of hemoglobin in the blood, which is very tightly correlated with the hct, so a doctor might just quote one of these numbers to a patient), and the platelet count. A patient who is puzzled by the numbers on the laboratory report should ask his or her doctor or nurse to explain them.

When someone is first diagnosed with leukemia, the doctor might obtain CBCs frequently, perhaps weekly or twice weekly, depending on the counts that are obtained. For example, if the patient's platelet or red blood cell counts are low enough to cause the doctor to consider need for blood or platelet transfusions (replacement of blood cells or platelets in the bloodstream when a person's own bone marrow is unable to do so), the frequency of blood draws will be higher.

Catheter, indwelling

Device placed surgically beneath the skin to facilitate the frequent infusion of medications and/ or other treatments (see port-a-cath).

Port-a-cath

A device surgically implanted under the skin, usually on the chest, that enters a large blood vessel and is used to deliver medication, chemotherapy, and blood products; also is used to obtain blood samples.

If a patient's veins are in good condition, this should not be difficult. However, some patients have more problems, and their blood draws become more difficult. Usually, before starting intense chemotherapy for acute leukemia or before a bone marrow transplantation, the patient will have a semi-permanent venous **catheter** surgically placed into one of the large veins under the collarbone or in the arm. Blood can be removed from this catheter for tests. In addition, medications and transfusions can be delivered through this intravenous catheter. This eliminates the need for repeated needle sticks in the veins, making the treatment process virtually painless for the patient and far easier for the nurses to complete. The actual catheter can be easily infected, so daily inspection and dressing changes are essential. Once the treatments are over, the frequency of CBCs and other blood tests will decline. The catheter can be removed in a same-day procedure when it no longer is needed as part of ongoing therapy. There are other venous access devices, including PIC lines and ports (small devices buried under the skin into which a needle can be used to withdraw blood or infuse medications or fluids). The choice of which venous access device is best for the patient is individualized and varies among medical centers.

17. What is a bone marrow biopsy/aspiration? Is it painful?

A **bone marrow biopsy/aspiration** is usually performed by a **hematologist** (a specialist in treating diseases, including malignancies, of the blood) or an **oncologist** (a specialist in **oncology**, the science dealing with the physical, chemical, and biologic properties and features of cancer, including causes, the disease process, and treatment). It involves inserting a needle into the cavity of the pelvis bone to withdraw samples of bone marrow and the surrounding bone. It is performed using local anesthesia (lidocaine) similar to what a dentist would use to work on a tooth. First, a needle is inserted into the bone marrow cavity to allow a small amount of liquid marrow (which looks like blood) to be withdrawn. After this needle is removed, a second needle is used to remove a small (about half an inch long) cylinder of bone, which then undergoes pathology testing (**biopsy**). The procedure takes about 30 minutes and is often considered uncomfortable. Of course, some patients experience more pain than others from this procedure, depending on their own sensitivity to pain, the skill of the person doing the procedure, and any technical difficulties encountered during the test. The purpose of the test is to examine cells in the bone marrow carefully under the microscope in order to determine whether any abnormalities exist. When leukemia is suspected, for example, based on an abnormality in the blood cells, it is necessary to do a bone marrow aspiration. This procedure might be repeated during leukemia treatment to monitor the progress of therapy. For example, after induction (initial) chemotherapy for leukemia, the bone marrow aspiration might be repeated to demonstrate that normal cells have repopulated the bone marrow and that the leukemia cells have been eliminated.

18. What are chromosomes/cytogenetics?

Every cell in the human body, with the exception of the red blood cells, contains a nucleus, which, in turn, contains

Bone marrow biopsy/aspiration

A procedure in which a needle is inserted into the center of a bone, usually the hip, to remove a small amount of bone marrow for microscopic examination.

Hematologist

A specialist who sees and treats patients with malignancies (and other diseases) of the blood.

Oncologist

A physician who specializes in cancer treatment.

Oncology

The science dealing with the physical, chemical and biologic properties and features of cancer, including causes, the disease process, and therapies.

Biopsy

Surgical removal of a small piece of tissue or a small tumor for microscopic examination to determine whether cancer cells are present. A biopsy is the most important procedure in diagnosing cancer.

chromosomes. The chromosomes are large, complex structures that contain DNA and proteins. The DNA (one of two types of nucleic acids, found in the nucleus of all cells) is organized into genes, which code for proteins that are necessary for all functionality of the cell and, ultimately, the individual. The anatomy of the chromosome can be studied by performing a clinical test called "karyotyping" or **cytogenetic analysis**. This analysis refers to a procedure whereby cells, taken from either the blood or the bone marrow, are cultured in a specialized laboratory in such a way that the dividing cells are arrested in the middle of their division. At this time, the chromosomes have organized themselves into structures that can be seen under the microscope with appropriate staining. In this manner, the number and the exact characteristics of the chromosomes can be seen. Normally, there are 46 chromosomes in each cell. A female has two X chromosomes and a male has an X and a Y chromosome. The remaining pairs of chromosomes do not differ according to gender. That is, chromosomes 1 through 22 are the same in a male or a female. In malignant cells, such as leukemia cells and lymphoma cells, unique alterations are observed on a regular basis in the chromosomes. Thus, cytogenetic analysis yields important information regarding the exact nature of the genetic defect that is associated with a given patient's leukemia. This, in turn, leads to important information regarding the patient's prognosis. For example, certain cytogenetic abnormalities, such as **translocations**, in which one piece of a chromosome moves to another chromosome, are associated with different prognoses after chemotherapy. Some abnormalities favor a good outcome—that is, chances are good that the patient will survive. Thus, the identification of one of these favorable cytogenetic abnormalities can lead to the application of the treatment that offers the best chance of survival without the excess risk posed by perhaps a more aggressive treatment.

Conversely, certain cytogenetic abnormalities have been associated with a very poor outcome. In such an event, a physician will use such information to consider not treating a patient aggressively, if the situation warrants this decision. For example, an elderly or infirm patient might be counseled to have supportive care or only mild chemotherapy if the prognosis is considered extremely poor, because chances are good that the treatment would not work and the patient would suffer a lower quality of life for no reason. The identification of these chromosomal changes has also been useful in leading to advances in the treatment of leukemia and in understanding more fundamental aspects of the biology of leukemia. It is considered routine to perform cytogenetic analysis on a newly diagnosed leukemia patient so that the prognosis can be determined.

In CML, a very characteristic and universal cytogenetic abnormality is observed. Under the microscope, one can see a very small piece of chromosomal material, originally called the **Philadelphia chromosome**, which results from a translocation of part of chromosome 9 to chromosome 22 and vice versa. This 9;22 translocation is diagnostic of CML; in other words, if the translocation is present, the doctor can be absolutely certain that the patient has CML.

The identification of the genes involved has also allowed the discovery of the **pathogenesis** (the origin and development) of this disease. The genes code for a recently identified protein referred to as "bcr/abl," which is responsible for the excess cellular division observed in CML. The abl portion of the molecule is an enzyme that acts to drive cellular proliferation. A designer drug was created to block the activity of this enzyme. This drug, imatinib mesylate (see Question 22), inhibits this enzyme, which is unique to CML. Subsequently, two additional drugs have been created, dasatinib and nilotinib, both of which are highly active and increasingly used to treat CML.

Cytogenetic analysis in ALL is useful in demonstrating that a large proportion (33%) of adult patients with ALL have the Philadelphia chromosome in their cells. This is an important observation because it is now established that the addition of one of the new treatments for CML improves the outcome

Thus, cytogenetic analysis yields important information regarding the exact nature of the genetic defect that is associated with a given patient's leukemia. This, in turn, leads to important information regarding the patient's prognosis.

Philadelphia chromosome

The abnormal chromosome found in patients with CML.

Pathogenesis

The origin and development of a disease.

of treatment for Philadelphia chromosome-positive ALL. Previously, the prognosis of patients with this type of ALL was quite poor compared with those without the translocation. This led to the use of bone marrow transplantation to patients with ALL who have the Philadelphia chromosome as the only curative therapy. At this time, the role of allogeneic transplantation is less clear and requires more research.

Patients with CLL frequently have an extra chromosome 12, referred to as "trisomy 12." This has been associated with a worse prognosis.

Cytogenetics are routinely performed at diagnosis in the acute leukemias and in suspected cases of CML. Cytogenetics might then be performed at different phases of treatment to document the elimination of these abnormal cells.

A supplement to cytogenetic testing is an even more refined type of test called molecular analysis. A number of specific molecular abnormalities have been identified in the genes of leukemia cells and many have significant prognostic significance. They are usually studied at the time of diagnosis and the results are then used in treatment planning, particularly in the decision to recommend a hematopoietic stem cell transplant.

19. What is immunophenotyping?

Growth factors

Substances that promote the growth of white blood cells.

Immunophenotyping

A laboratory test whereby an area's antigens can be measured on the surface of the leukemia cell.

Leukemia cells, like all blood cells, display numerous protein, carbohydrate, and lipid molecules on the outer surface of the cell. These various molecules, sometimes referred to as antigens, are often important components of the cell for signaling, attaching to surfaces, and as docking sites for **growth factors** for the leukemia or normal cells. **Immunophenotyping** refers to a laboratory test whereby these antigens can be measured on the surface of the leukemia cell. The purpose of this test is to determine the type of leukemia that exists in a given patient. For example, AML expresses antigens that are characteristic of normal granulocytes and monocytes, whereas ALL has the same antigens expressed by normal lymphocytes. A more refined application of this technique also involves identifying an abnormal immunophenotype, which can be used to monitor the progress of treatment. For example, a leukemia cell can express myeloid antigens predominantly but can also express a lymphoid antigen; however, this is not a normal situation. This mixed phenotype will then be monitored during treatment by repeating the immunophenotyping. The testing can be performed on blood cells as well as on bone marrow cells.

PART THREE

Treatment

How is leukemia treated?

What is chemotherapy?

How does my doctor decide which
chemotherapy to give me?

More . . .

20. How is leukemia treated?

Leukemia is a systemic disease, which means that any treatment administered must be able to reach all parts of the body. There is no role for surgery and a very, very limited role for **radiation therapy** (treatment with high-energy X-rays to destroy cancer cells). Thus, therapy for leukemia consists of the administration of chemotherapy. Chemotherapy is more or less defined as therapy with **cytotoxic drugs**, that is, drugs that are able to kill leukemia cells. A large number of drugs that are specific for the different forms of leukemia are used to treat it. Other approaches to the treatment of leukemia include immunotherapy, which involves using monoclonal antibodies, certain types of cells, or certain biologic molecules referred to as cytokines, such as interleukin-2 (see Question 28). Many of these therapies are investigational at this time.

A patient with acute leukemia who has achieved a complete remission but has a high probability of relapse might undergo a **hematopoietic stem cell transplantation** (provision of new stem cells to the patient) to improve the odds of staying in complete remission (see Question 33).

21. What is chemotherapy?

Chemotherapy refers to the administration of drugs that are capable of killing cancer cells, or at least retarding their growth. These drugs are manufactured by the pharmaceutical industry and are regulated by the FDA, whose approval is required for their commercial use. Chemotherapy drugs may be given **orally** (by mouth, e.g., imatinib mesylate, hydroxyurea), **intravenously** (injected into a vein, e.g., cytosine arabinoside, fludarabine), or even **subcutaneously** (injected under the skin, e.g., L-asparaginase). Chemotherapy has been the mainstay of leukemia treatment for decades. Recently, biologic agents, such as monoclonal antibodies (see Question 27), are increasingly used either alone or in conjunction with conventional chemotherapy.

Radiation therapy

Treatment with high-energy X-rays to destroy cancer cells.

Cytotoxic

Drugs that can kill cancer cells. Usually refers to drugs used in chemotherapy treatments.

Hematopoietic stem cell transplantation

The process by which new stem cells are introduced into a patient.

Chemotherapy

Treatment of cancer by use of chemicals; often uses two or more chemicals to achieve maximum kill of tumor cells. Usually refers to drugs used to treat cancer.

Orally

Taken by mouth.

Intravenously

Entering the body through a vein.

Subcutaneously

Injected under the skin.

Table 1 lists some of the medications used to treat leukemia. The exact treatment of an individual takes many factors into consideration. There is no single drug or combination that is considered so standard that every doctor uses it. The names of medications can be confusing—drugs can be referred to by their trade (brand) name or by their generic name. Furthermore, sometimes an abbreviated slang-like use will be employed. For example, the drug cytosine arabinoside (generic) may be called cytarabine (another generic), Cytosar-U (trade), or ara-c (slang). Obviously, this can be confusing to the patient. Patients who are confused about what they are hearing should ask their doctors to clarify!

22. What is a tyrosine kinase inhibitor?

Tyrosine kinase inhibitors are a general class of drugs that work by blocking the action of one or more of the many enzymes called tyrosine kinases that promote growth of leukemia cells. The first in class was **Gleevec**, the trade name for a chemical called imatinib mesylate. In the clinical trial phase of its development, this drug was also called STI–571. Imatinib mesylate is a small chemical molecule that was developed to specifically inhibit the enzyme that is overactive in patients with CML. The malignant cells in CML have an abnormal protein that has heightened activity of a particular tyrosine kinase called abl. Imatinib mesylate inhibits the enzyme so that its activity is suppressed in the CML cells. Doctors and patients alike were pleasantly surprised by the findings that this oral drug could give rise to remissions in CML. At one level, the remission is called **hematologic**, meaning that the blood counts return to normal. More importantly, some patients experience a disappearance of the Philadelphia chromosome, which means that there is even less likelihood of the disease coming right back. This is called a **cytogenetic remission**.

Finally, some patients even achieve **molecular remissions**, in which special tests that can amplify very small numbers of cells can be used to see whether the disease has been totally eradicated.

Gleevec
Oral chemotherapy agent approved for use in patients with CML.

Hematologic remission
Remission defined by the blood counts' return to normal.

Cytogenetic remission
Remission defined by the chromosomes in the bone marrow cells returning to normal with no evidence of the Philadelphia chromosome.

Molecular remission
Remission defined by analysis of small numbers of cells that indicate that a disease is totally eradicated.

The FDA approved imatinib mesylate in 2001 for CML patients. It has been quite safe, with the only serious side effects being fluid retention, rash, hemorrhage, bleeding, and kidney and liver toxicity, and those in only a small number of patients. Most patients tolerate imatinib mesylate very well without any side effects. Because the drug has not been in use for many years, it is impossible to predict its long-term effectiveness. Some believe that patients with the most profound decrease in their malignant cells (whose disease cannot be detected even with molecular techniques) will experience long-term survival without recurrence of the disease. Patients who have more accelerated or blastic forms of CML also respond, but their responses are temporary. Thus, this drug is increasingly used to treat the more aggressive forms of CML temporarily while arrangements are attempted for a bone marrow transplant.

The role of bone marrow transplantation for patients in the first chronic phase of CML is declining. While it is widely recognized that stem cell transplantation is the only known curative therapy for CML, tyrosine kinase inhibitors have been shown to be so effective that transplantation is now considered a second-line therapy for most patients.

Two other tyrosine kinase inhibitors have been approved by the FDA. One is dasatinib (trade name: Sprycel), approved by the FDA in 2006 for the treatment of imatinib mesylate-resistant CML and for Philadelphia chromosome-positive ALL and then later approved for initial treatment of chronic phase CML. In addition, nilotinib (trade name: Tasigna), was initially approved by the FDA in 2007 for accelerated phase CML and then for initial treatment of chronic phase CML in 2010. Unfortunately, neither of the three approved tyrosine kinase inhibitors are effective when a certain mutation occurs in the genes in CML cells. A mutation called T315I makes the CML cells resistant to therapy in a small percentage of patients. There is a need for a more effective medicine for this situation. A drug called ponatinib is in development but is currently considered experimental and not available outside of clinical trials.

23. What is ATRA? How can arsenic be a treatment for leukemia?

ATRA stands for all-trans-retinoic acid, a drug whose structure is related to that of vitamin A. Amazingly, this drug, which was first studied by Chinese doctors, induces the relatively uncommon form of AML known as promyelocytic leukemia (which accounts for 10% of AML diagnoses) to differentiate into normal end-stage white blood cells. This means that the leukemic cells become like normal white blood cells, so the effects of leukemia disappear. Another bonus is that this drug is given orally. However, because ATRA alone does not produce long-lasting remissions, current treatment protocols combine ATRA with conventional anti-AML drugs, such as idarubicin (Idamycin) or daunorubicin (Cerubidine).

Arsenic trioxide, also discovered by Chinese scientists, is able to induce differentiation in promyelocytic leukemia cells as well. It is now approved by the FDA for use in patients with relapsed promyelocytic leukemia, and it is also being tested in clinical trials against other types of cancer. Recent studies continue to show the importance of arsenic trioxide in the treatment of APL, possible even as initial therapy.

24. How does my doctor decide which chemotherapy to give me?

This is a very complicated question, and standards of care for leukemia are evolving continually. A large amount of clinical research has gone into the creation of the current treatment protocols. However, because none of the current treatments are perfect, clinical research and clinical trials continue to seek better treatments. In addition, new **pharmaceuticals** (medications) are always being developed, which allows the introduction of these new agents into treatment protocols. So how your doctor decides to treat your leukemia has a lot to do with who your doctor is, the type of medical center in which you are being treated, the specifics of your illness, your age, and other potential health problems. Relatively standard treatments for

Pharmaceuticals
Medications that are continuously being developed for future patient care.

each of the major leukemias do exist, but there is constant evolution in the treatments because the perfect treatment that can cure everyone has not yet been discovered.

You might be offered entry into a clinical trial at a major medical center (see Question 29). Clinical trials have been carefully considered and reviewed by multiple levels of scrutiny and are believed to offer the best chance of remission and long-term survival. However, the requirements for entry into a clinical trial are fairly rigid. Therefore, it is not uncommon for a patient to be treated with a standard regimen instead of being entered into a clinical trial. This is where the experience of your physician and his or her institution are relevant. For example, one institution might be very comfortable giving one form of therapy, while another institution might be more comfortable with a different form of therapy, which its staff believes is equally effective. This can be difficult for you to sort out and understand. Further decision making hinges on your physician's assessment of your disease and your overall condition. For instance, if you are an older patient with other problems, such as heart failure or coronary artery disease, you might be treated less aggressively than you would be if you were a young patient with no preexisting illness. Finally, the use of **prognostic factors**, such as cytogenetics, could direct treatment to be more or less aggressive. It is not unreasonable to ask your physician to explain his or her thinking regarding the choice of treatments offered to you for any form of leukemia.

Clinical trials have been carefully considered and reviewed by multiple levels of scrutiny and are believed to offer the best chance of remission and long-term survival.

Prognostic factors

Factors that help to determine the severity of a disease.

Protocol

A schedule of selected drugs and treatment time intervals known to be effective against a certain cancer.

The **protocols** (schedules of drugs and treatment) for treating the different types of leukemia vary. Protocols are constantly changing, and new drugs are becoming available constantly. However, with new medications can come undiscovered challenges. Each person has different reactions, because each of our chemistries is unique. Even though the chemotherapy drugs are generally safe, there is an unavoidable risk of side effects, and you should be made aware of potential side effects that might occur either immediately or later. You should also inquire whether there are any interactions between your chemotherapy drugs and any other medications you might be taking.

25. What is gene therapy? What are chimeric antigen receptors?

Gene therapy is a term applied to a wide range of research efforts to introduce new genetic material into cells in order to modify their DNA. There have been some intriguing early successes in the use of this therapeutic approach for patients with immune deficiency states and hemophilia. However, in general, this is still a very investigational form of therapy. Applications in leukemia would include efforts to render leukemia cells more antigenic (meaning foreign) to the immune system of the patient. Other efforts might be to introduce genes into the chromosomes that decrease the proliferative rate of leukemia cells.

An intriguing new approach to gene therapy involves the creation of killer T cells that have a targeting molecule similar to an antibody that can seek out leukemia cells bearing the target of the antibody-like molecule. This promising technique, involving the use of chimeric antigen receptors (CARs), could allow potent antileukemia therapy of many leukemia patients. However it is important to note that at the time this book went to press, this is still a highly experimental technique and is only available at a very select group of research institutions that are studying this method. Studies are ongoing that will determine if this is an effective and safe therapy.

26. What is antisense therapy?

Antisense therapy is another investigational therapy for a variety of diseases, including leukemia and other forms of cancer. The basic idea of antisense therapy is to block the production of a key protein involved in the progression of a cancer using specially crafted strings of DNA that can get into cells and block the corresponding RNA that makes the

Gene therapy
Investigational treatment of disease by the introduction of new genetic material into cells in order to modify their DNA.

Antisense therapy
Emerging investigational therapy for various diseases that blocks protein production.

protein of interest. The protein that the cancer cell makes is made by the sense strand of RNA. The antisense is the mirror image of the sense strand and is able to neutralize it. For example, leukemia cells have an excess of a protein called bcl-2 that blocks the normal death of a cell. Blocking bcl-2 production leads to death of leukemia cells in the laboratory. Clinical trials of bcl-2 antisense are being conducted to determine whether a therapeutic benefit can be achieved in patients with AML and other cancers. Clinical trials of antisense targeting the p53 gene are also under way.

27. What is a monoclonal antibody?

Monoclonal antibody

Antibody that specifically binds to a particular molecule on the surface of a certain type of leukemia or other cancer.

Molecule

The smallest particle of a substance that retains the properties of the substance; composed of one or more atoms.

A **monoclonal antibody** is a highly specialized antibody that is usually produced initially by immunizing a mouse with an antigen of interest. The spleen from the mouse is then fused with a cell type that lends the property of immortality to the lymphocytes in the spleen. This cell, known as a hybridoma, produces an unlimited quantity of a single antibody **molecule** from the lymphocyte. This antibody is known as a monoclonal antibody (which is an antibody with only one specificity or antigen). Research scientists have employed this process for more than 20 years since its discovery by the Nobel prize winners Koehler and Milstein. Recently, because of the ability to produce human monoclonal antibodies, the human forms have replaced the mouse antibodies in clinical trials. These human monoclonal antibodies can be produced such that they specifically bind to a particular molecule on the surface of a certain type of leukemia or other cancer. Thus, monoclonal antibodies are available to antigens expressed on leukemia cells that either are now approved for clinical use or are under active study in clinical trials. For example, gemtuzumab ozogamicin (Mylotarg), a monoclonal antibody with a chemotherapy drug attached to it, was approved by the FDA, but the approval was withdrawn for various reasons, thus making it now an investigational agent. Another monoclonal antibody, alemtuzumab (Campath), was also approved for the treatment of CLL. The monoclonal antibodies rituxumab (Rituxan) and ofatumumab (Arzerra) are also increasingly used to treat CLL. Many more monoclonal antibodies are under active study and hopefully will be available for wide use in the future. It is expected that the optimal use of monoclonal antibodies will *usually* be in combination with standard chemotherapy agents, providing therapies that are more potent without being more toxic.

28. What is immunotherapy?

Immunotherapy is a general term referring to the use of the immune system to treat disease. There has been an interest in immunotherapy for a long time, based on theory and animal studies that the immune system itself can control tumor growth. However, most immunotherapeutic approaches to the treatment of leukemia remain investigational. That said, there are now a number of emerging immunotherapies that seem to be effective. In the treatment of leukemia, immunotherapy could mean the use of monoclonal antibodies, cytokines such as interleukin-2, or cells such as T lymphocytes and natural killer cells. Immunotherapy is considered to be a biologic therapy because it harnesses normal components of our bodies in an effort to direct these elements to help eliminate the leukemia. Considerable interest was aroused by a recent study where investigators inserted specially created receptors into killer T cells that could target leukemia cells, resulting in good clinical responses and ongoing effects by the genetically-altered cells. (See Gene Therapy, Question 25).

Immunotherapy
Treatment that stimulates the body's own defense mechanisms to combat diseases such as cancer.

29. What is a clinical trial?

A **clinical trial** is a study examining the safety and effectiveness of a treatment of an illness. There are many kinds of clinical trials, and therefore it is important to understand the distinction between them.

A phase I clinical trial is the earliest testing of a new drug or the use of an established drug for a different disease. For example, a drug might already be approved for treating a certain form of leukemia, but it might be tested for the treatment of a different form of leukemia in a phase I study that is trying to determine the safety and the best dose of the drug for the second form of leukemia.

Clinical trial
A form of clinical research where patients are treated on carefully designed regimens of drugs to determine their safety and efficacy.

Treatment

A phase II study typically involves the use of a particular drug at a fixed dose, which has been already established in a phase I study to be safe and possibly effective. The phase II study attempts to determine the effectiveness of the drug used in a standard manner in a larger number of patients.

A phase III study typically compares the activity of one drug or combination of drugs with the activity of another drug or combination of drugs, both of which are already established as having activity in a particular disease. The phase III study might determine whether a new drug or combination of drugs that has recently been developed can be more effective than the established treatment for that particular leukemia. Clinical trials are sometimes referred to as *investigational* or *experimental*. These terms sometimes cause confusion, especially when it comes to payment for treatment by insurance companies; many insurance companies have clauses that deny coverage for the use of experimental treatments for their members. However, in the treatment of leukemia, a drug that has shown promise but has not yet received FDA approval might be used. Thus, an insurance company might state that the treatment is experimental and might therefore deny coverage, even when the community of physicians has determined that this could be the best new drug for leukemia in some time. An insurance company might even deem it experimental when an FDA-approved drug is included in a clinical trial if it is used in a slightly different dose or schedule, again with the goal of improving outcomes.

Experts in leukemia treatment are always trying to improve the outcomes of treatment, but they sometimes get caught in a bind with the third-party payers of the treatment. Frequently, when truly experimental agents, such as new drugs, are being used, the sponsoring pharmaceutical company pays for all elements of the treatment that are considered investigational. This would include the drug itself and any additional testing that would be performed specifically because the patient was in a clinical trial. Certain legislation has been enacted to mandate that insurance companies pay for treatment that oc-curs in clinical trials, recognizing that advances in treatment can come only from widespread participation in clinical tri-als. It is notable that in pediatric populations, approximately 95% of patients in the United States are treated in national-level clinical trials. In contrast, only 5% of adult patients are enrolled in clinical trials in the United States. Studies have shown that outcomes in patient care are improved when pa-tients are treated in clinical trials, presumably because of the intense scrutiny involved when the patient is treated in a clini-cal trial. Clinical trial monitoring is very intense and rigorous, and this increased attention to the details of management, quality of life, follow-up, and compliance with treatment are probable reasons for improved outcomes in clinical trials.

30. What are study drugs? Are there any promising new drugs in development?

Clinical trials may consist of studies of new agents. Therefore, a study drug is a new pharmacologic agent that is being tested for a new therapeutic activity. The usual course of events is that new agents are discovered in academic or pharmaceutical laboratories and that these agents have activity on leukemia cells in the laboratory. For example, a drug that kills leukemia cells in the test tube might be identified. After appropriate safety testing in small animal strains and possibly even in primates (that is, monkeys and apes, which are the animals most closely related to humans), the drug is then introduced to patients who have advanced disease. After efficacy and safety are shown, the drug is then pursued in more widespread clinical trials.

As of the publication of this book, several new drugs are in development for the treatment of leukemia. Current thinking is that successful drugs need to target the abnormal proteins in leukemia cells that are responsible for making the cells grow in such an uncontrolled manner. Two of these are inves-tigational drugs that target selected biochemical pathways in acute leukemia cells that are abnormally activated to promote leukemia cell growth. These drugs target the enzyme farnesyl transferase and the cell surface protein FLT–3, two proteins involved in the control of cell division. In addition, a class of drugs that can inhibit the enzyme histone deacetylase is under study. This inhibition results in the removal of gene-silencing molecules that somehow contribute to leukemia cell growth. Other targets for antileukemia therapy include angiogenesis inhibitors, including thalidomide and lenalidomide, SU5416, hypomethylating agents such as 5-azacytidine and decitabine, and monoclonal antibodies to vascular endothelial growth factor, with the hope that attacking the blood supply to leukemia cells will starve them to death.

The new drugs might also work better in combination with established chemotherapy agents.

These approaches are all investigational. Some of the drugs will work; others won't. In addition, certain drugs might work on certain leukemias and not on other leukemias. The new drugs might also work better in combination with established chemotherapy agents. Patients should ask their doctors about what clinical trials are available, whether at their doctor's institution or practice or elsewhere.

31. What determines who is eligible for a study?

A clinical trial has strict eligibility and exclusion criteria for entry into the study; the exact diagnosis, subtypes of leukemia, age of the patient, history of previous treatment, history of other illnesses, and a myriad of other issues are addressed in these criteria. However, the physician or the patient must first be aware of the clinical trials. This crucial step is often lacking and is the reason many patients are not enrolled in clinical trials. Once it is recognized that a patient might be eligible for a particular clinical trial, there are numerous support staff at large institutions or at clinical trial-oriented private practices that are available for screening patients for eligibility. In addition to obvious factors, such as diagnosis, age, and type of leukemia, a number of laboratory tests will be performed to determine that the overall health of the patient is suited for the study. The process of **informed consent** is always utilized. This means that the patient is told explicitly what the elements of the clinical trial are and what the risks and benefits to the patient could be. The patient may withdraw from treatment at any time, because participation in the study is completely voluntary. The patient signs an agreement to the terms of the study. This so-called consent form is then part of the patient's medical record.

Informed consent

Process of explanation to the patient of all risks and complications of a procedure or treatment before it is done. Most informed consents are written and signed by the patient or a legal representative

Treatment

PART FOUR

Blood and Marrow Stem Cell Transplantation

What is a stem cell?

What is stem cell transplantation?

Who should have a stem cell transplant?

More . . .

32. What is a stem cell?

Broadly defined, a **stem cell** is a type of cell in the body that can continuously replenish the cells of that particular **tissue** (a tissue is a collection of similar cells). One can think of it as a seed that gives rise to the remainder of cells in that particular tissue. This implies that there are organ-specific stem cells. For example, there is a type of stem cell that resides in the bone marrow that is capable of giving rise to all of the blood cells that are first formed in the bone marrow and then travel to the blood. This cell is referred to as a **hematopoietic stem cell**. There appear to be stem cells in other organs as well, which are specific for those organs. For instance, there could be a liver (hepatic) stem cell, a muscle stem cell, and a neural stem cell. There are also intriguing observations suggesting that stem cells from one tissue can actually still retain some properties of giving rise to cells of another tissue under certain conditions. This is referred to as "stem cell plasticity." A general property of stem cells is that they can renew themselves. Thus, when a stem cell divides, it replenishes itself, but it also gives rise to a daughter cell that begins the process of differentiation into the tissues in which it resides. Stem cells are rare in any tissue. They make up no more than 0.01% of the total cells in the bone marrow, for example. They can be defined with certain cell-surface markers and by their abilities to make colonies of blood cells in the laboratory. The bone marrow stem cell can migrate into the blood. These are the cells that are transplanted in a bone marrow transplant.

33. What is stem cell transplantation?

The term **stem cell transplantation** has crept into the jargon of medicine. Previously, these treatments were referred to as "bone marrow transplants" or BMTs. In a BMT, the goal is to transplant the hematopoietic stem cell. In general, stem cell transplantation is the process by which stem cells are infused into a patient. The patient is generally prepared for the procedure by administration of very high doses of chemotherapy in a hospital setting over a period of several days, with careful monitoring and adjustment of the chemotherapy. Before receiving chemotherapy, the patient usually has an indwelling catheter placed (see Question 16), allowing for easier administration of chemotherapy, blood drawing, blood transfusions, and antibiotic therapy.

Recovery can be slow because the stem cells have to begin producing blood cells again. When that happens (after a period of weeks), the patient is most fragile and is at high risk for infection. Extreme caution and careful management of food, diet, dust, and exposure to elements, as well as limiting of visitors, will enhance the patient's ability to successfully navigate this difficult period until the blood counts recover.

34. Who should have a stem cell transplant?

This is a complicated question that requires considerable deliberation and judgment by the patient and the doctor alike. Stem cell transplants have been commonly used in the management of the acute leukemias and CML. That said, only a small fraction of patients with these forms of leukemia end up getting a stem cell transplant. The goal of transplantation is usually cure. Those making the decision must consider the odds that a cure could be achieved by conventional chemotherapy, compared with the odds that a transplant will achieve that goal. Several factors are considered, including the age of the patient, the molecular characteristics of the disease, and the availability of a suitable stem cell **donor** (one who donates cells or marrow). To some extent, the decision to undergo transplantation can be subjected to objective criteria that can even be reduced to an algorithm. For example, a patient with AML under the age of 60 who has an HLA-matched sibling donor (see Question 46) and whose disease has features that predict a poor prognosis with standard therapy would most likely have allogeneic stem cell transplantation recommended. On the other hand, if a patient's leukemia has good risk features, meaning that his or her prognosis looks favorable, allogeneic stem cell transplantation might not offer

Donor

One who donates blood stem cells or bone marrow for infusion into a patient.

an increased chance of cure, and therefore, the increased risk of transplantation is not warranted. As new information is generated from clinical research studies, the decision of who should undergo transplantation requires careful and considered judgment. Patients should ask their doctors to explain why they should or shouldn't be referred for a blood or bone marrow stem cell transplant.

35. What is the difference between autologous and allogeneic transplantation?

Autologous stem cell transplantation involves the use of cells from the patient's own body. Blood stem cells are generally collected by use of a special intravenous catheter placed directly either into a vein in the arm or under the collarbone. Autologous stem cell transplantations are commonly used in leukemia, lymphoma, and myeloma. The patient must be in remission so that stem cells that are not contaminated with cancer cells can be collected. Allogeneic stem cell transplantation involves the use of cells from someone other than the patient. Typically, a sibling donor who is matched at histocompatibility antigens (see Question 46) is called on to donate either bone marrow or blood stem cells to be infused into the patient, who has received chemotherapy or radiotherapy to prepare for the stem cell transplant. Recently, doctors are trying less intense chemotherapy or radiation doses in an effort to reduce the toxicity of allogeneic stem cell transplantation. These transplants have been referred to as *mini transplants, reduced intensity transplants,* or *non-myeloablative transplants*—all terms referring to the same concept. Occasionally, a patient has an identical twin who could act as a donor. The advantage of this situation is that the donor and the patient are fully matched for all important tissue antigens. Thus, there is no expected graft-versus-host reaction (see Questions 62–64) or rejection. The only disadvantage is that there is also less of a graft-versus-leukemia effect (see Question 63), because the donor lymphocytes do not recognize any of the patient's leukemia cell antigens as foreign. Unrelated donors that are well matched with the patient are also used for allogeneic transplants.

Another form of unrelated donor cells is from umbilical cord blood, and there are numerous cord blood registries now that might have a suitably matched unit, stored frozen, already in the bank. There is less experience with this form of transplant for adults, but the number of transplantations performed with umbilical cord blood is increasing.

36. How is it determined which type of transplant is appropriate for my care?

The decision of whether to perform autologous versus alloge-neic transplantation is complicated. The first issue is whether there is a suitable donor for you. If there is not a sibling or closely related family member who is matched at the histo-compatibility antigens (see Question 46), allogeneic stem cell transplantation is ruled out. An unrelated donor transplanta-tion might be pursued, but given the higher rates of graft-versus-host disease (GVHD, see Questions 62–64) with this type of transplantation, it is limited to a younger population of patients—generally under 50, but now perhaps up to 75 years of age with reduced-intensity preparative regimens for allogeneic transplants. Autologous transplantation is used in some cases of acute leukemia, based on clinical trials that have shown the relative value of these transplants. Your age and overall physical condition are factors in the decision of which type of transplantation to pursue, as are some of the characteristics of the disease. Of course, if there is not a suit-able HLA-matched donor, then an autologous transplanta-tion is your only transplant option.

37. How long after diagnosis should a transplant take place?

This, again, is a complex clinical decision. If an HLA-matched sibling is available for a patient with acute leukemia in first complete remission, there is evidence that proceeding to transplantation after achieving this complete remission is often the best course of action. Ideally, the patient should have recovered fully from the effects of chemotherapy and not have any lingering side effects or infections before undergoing the bone marrow transplantation. If a decision had already been made not to do the transplantation in first remission and the patient eventually has a relapse, then transplantation should be strongly considered after a second remission is induced.

Transplants were formerly the treatment of choice in CML in the first year after diagnosis. The discovery of the drug imatinib mesylate (Gleevec) and similar drugs have led most patients to try these drugs first and forgo transplantation unless a remission isn't achieved or they have a relapse.

38. What is total body irradiation (TBI)? Will I need to have it?

Allogeneic transplantation for AML, ALL, and CML often includes total body irradiation (TBI). There is an alternative regimen that involves drugs only. TBI means that the entire body is exposed to the same intensity of radiation. Radiation physicians and physicists carefully calculate the dose, so that the amount of radiation getting into every part of the body is approximately the same. This is important because leukemia cells can be dispersed throughout every capillary and blood vessel in the body, so it is necessary to irradiate the entire body to ensure that every leukemia cell is irradiated. The radiation is delivered in several sessions over a few days to minimize side effects.

39. What are immunosuppressive drugs, and who is likely to need them?

Patients undergoing stem cell transplantation from a donor (allogeneic transplantation) require treatment with immunosuppressive drugs. This is because if the function of the patient's immune system is not suppressed, the transplanted donor cells would be immediately rejected. Immunosuppression allows the transplanted donor cells to survive and eventually develop the new bone marrow and immune system. Another reason that immunosuppressive drugs are used in this type of transplantation is that they decrease the likelihood of graft-versus-host disease (see Questions 62–64). The immunosuppressive drugs decrease the aggressiveness of the newly developing immune system, which might react against the patient's tissues if the immunosuppressive drugs were not being given.

Many drugs are immunosuppressive; the most familiar immunosuppressive drug to many patients is prednisone, or its intravenous form, solumedrol. Dexamethasone (Decadron) is another variation of prednisone that is commonly used for immunosuppression. Other drugs often used, including cyclosporine (Neoral) and tacrolimus (FK–506, Prograf), are very selective inhibitors of T-lymphocyte function, whereas prednisone has broader actions on a variety of cells and tissues in the body. The side effects of prednisone and its relatives are numerous and include high blood sugar, thinning of the bones, mood changes, and deterioration of muscle tissue. All of these side effects are dose and time dependent, meaning that if a patient has to receive high doses of the drug for a longer period of time, the side effects are much more likely to occur. On the other hand, if the drugs are used for a brief period of time, the side effects might be minimal. Side effects of cyclosporine and tacrolimus are somewhat different. These agents sometimes cause mild kidney failure, high blood pressure, and neurologic side effects, such as vision changes and seizures. Again, these side effects, although serious, are uncommon, and they are dose and time dependent.

Another important side effect of immunosuppressive drugs is an increased incidence of infection. Because the immune system is depressed, patients are likely to develop any of the

All of these side effects are dose and time dependent, meaning that if a patient has to receive high doses of the drug for a longer period of time, the side effects are much more likely to occur.

infections that will be discussed later (see Question 56). Doctors take this into consideration when using immunosuppressive drugs. They might place their patients on prophylactic antibiotics (therapy geared to prevent infection) to decrease the chance that an infection will develop. On balance, the benefits from these drugs far exceed the side effects.

40. Do I need to stay on immunosuppressive drugs for life?

The answer is generally, "no." Usually, a patient's tolerance of the graft develops in the first 6 to 12 months after transplant, leading to the opportunity to withdraw immune suppression. Occasionally, chronic graft-versus-host disease (see Question 64) will require prolonged immunosuppression, sometimes for life. The degree of immunosuppression can be quite variable between patients, ranging from very mild, such as a small dose of prednisone, to more intense multidrug regimens.

41. How soon will I regain my immune system after transplantation?

Immunodeficiency after stem cell transplantation is common and prolonged. If you have an HLA-matched sibling transplantation (see Question 46), your immune system will probably return to normal after approximately 1 year. If you undergo unrelated donor stem cell transplantation, the immunodeficiency might last for a longer period of time because the new T cells are not able to react to antigens as well in this situation.

42. What is the success rate of bone marrow transplantation?

People often want to know the answer to this general question, but it is difficult to give a simple answer. The main reason for this is that the answer differs for each type of leukemia, and it is also dependent on the age of the patient, the time in the history of the disease at which the transplantation is performed, and the type of transplantation performed. A very general answer is that approximately 50% of the patients who undergo a bone marrow transplantation will be alive 5 years later. Some groups of patients do have much better outcomes, such as patients with CML in the first chronic phase undergoing a transplant from a sibling donor. On the other hand, older patients undergoing unrelated donor transplantation for acute leukemia in late remissions, such as a second or third remission, might only have a 20% survival rate after 5 years.

The reasons for an undesirable outcome are toxicity from the regimen, severe GVHD, or relapse of the underlying disease. Each of these three events occurs for different reasons, and they vary between patients and the different diseases. It is best for each patient to discuss with his or her own doctor what the odds are for his or her specific situation. Regardless of the statistics quoted, the thing to keep in mind is that the expectation is for a better outcome with the transplant than without it.

BONE MARROW DONOR OR BLOOD STEM CELL DONOR

43. How long does it take to get a donor?

If a doctor recommends an allogeneic BMT, the choices of donor include siblings; other related donors, such as parents and children; and unrelated but matched donors. The process of HLA testing is relatively quick. After blood samples are obtained from the patient and potential donors, the determination of whether a match is available takes only 1 to 2 weeks. If a more extensive search for an unrelated donor must take place, the time required to identify and confirm a donor's eligibility takes up to several months. The initial process consists of a computer check for how many potential donors exist in the national registry. When potential donors are identified, further laboratory testing must be done on samples to determine whether the match is a full match or a partial match; this process can take 1 to 2 months. A potential donor must be cleared medically by his or her physician to be a stem cell donor. The stem cell donor is required to either have a **bone marrow harvest** under general anesthesia in the operating room or, increasingly common, to have peripheral blood stem cells collected in a process called **apheresis**.

Apheresis involves receiving a growth factor such as **granulocyte colony-stimulating factor** (G-CSF, a growth factor given to activate production of cells) by injection for several days, followed by the placement of an intravenous catheter to remove blood for the purpose of filtering the blood on a cell separation device. The donor reclines in a collection chair while the blood is removed and centrifuged to remove the fraction of cells that contain stem cells. This process takes several hours daily for 1 to 3 days. The collection is stopped when it is determined that sufficient stem cells were obtained.

44. If I have an unrelated donor transplantation, do I get to meet the donor?

The current rules and regulations used by the **National Marrow Donor Program** (NMDP) are that the identity of an unrelated donor is confidential in the first year after transplantation. After this, the identity of the donor can be revealed. Frequently, attempts are made by the donor and recipient to meet personally and share experiences and celebrate. This can be a very emotional experience for both the donor and the recipient, as well as their families.

45. Where do the donors come from?

The NMDP is one of several large registries with several million potential donors in its files. Donors have volunteered to have their blood typed for the availability of a stem cell transplant in the future. Many donors have come forward during blood drives or to answer the needs of a family member or a

---

Bone marrow harvest

Under general anesthesia, marrow is collected for later infusion into the patient.

Apheresis

The process of having peripheral blood stem cells collected.

Granulocyte colony-stimulating factor

Growth factors given to activate production of cells.

National Marrow Donor Program

A large registry with millions of potential donors in its files for future stem cell transplants.

particular patient of whom they are aware. Donors are literally everywhere in the world, and the American NMDP registry can tap into international registries. Currently, there are over 14 million potential donors registered in the NMDP and other worldwide registries. Hematopoietic stem cells, bone marrow, or blood are collected at the site where the donor has registered. The cells are flown to the transplant center where the patient will undergo the transplantation.

The process of infusing the donor stem cells into the hospitalized patient through an intravenous line takes from 1 to several hours. It is almost always uneventful, but minor (and reversible) allergic reactions can take place, similar to those in blood transfusions. The patient is always carefully observed during the stem cell infusion process, which can seem anticlimactic after all the preparation, chemotherapy, and testing that has led up to this important time.

46. Is a sibling or family member always the best donor choice?

The answer is almost always, "yes." However, **HLA-matched siblings** must be perfectly matched at the histocompatibility antigens currently tested. If the sibling is not matched for at least five of the six major antigens, then an alternative donor might be the best choice. Some transplantations are performed using children of the patient or a parent of the patient as the donor. Almost always, there is significant mismatching in this situation, but if only one or two antigens are mismatched, this might still be the patient's best option. Although this is a less-than-optimal situation, many successful transplants have been performed in this manner.

HLA-matched sibling

Compatible sister or brother who is determined by testing to be matched at specific loci.

47. Is a young donor better than an older one?

This is a complicated question. In general, a young donor is probably superior to an older donor within some limits. Between the ages of 20 and 50, there is probably not that much difference between donors. It might be difficult to obtain stem cells from older donors in particular, such as those over 60. However, typically, if a donor is young, that would mean that the patient is probably young as well, given that the age range of most full siblings is usually not more than 15 to 20 years. And usually, the age range is much less; thus, a sibling donor is likely to be close to the same age as the patient. Thus, outcomes of such transplantations are much more related to the age of the patient than that of the donor.

Outcomes of such trans-plantations are much more re-lated to the age of the patient than that of the donor.

48. Does my blood type change after BMT?

The red cell blood type changes to that of the donor after BMT. That means that if you have blood type A before transplantation and the donor is blood type O, eventually you will end up with blood type O. It can take several weeks to months for the type A blood cells to totally disappear, but they eventually will. Occasionally, after transplantation in the situation just described, antibodies formed by the donor lymphocytes destroy the red blood cells of the recipient of type A. This can sometimes cause clinical problems, such as pain and rapid red blood cell destruction with severe anemia. Usually, however, the process is relatively silent and benign. The histocompatibility antigens (**human leukocyte antigens**, HLAs) of the blood cells also change after allogeneic transplantation. The donor cells will engraft, and all blood cells then take on the HLA identity of the donor.

Human leukocyte antigen

The protein on the surface of all cells that must be matched for bone marrow transplants.

49. Can I be an organ donor after transplantation? How about a blood donor?

A diagnosis of cancer excludes you from being either an organ donor or a blood donor. Therefore, even if the leukemia has been cured, the need for extreme caution in maintaining a safe blood supply as well as the need to do no harm to a potential organ recipient dictates that as a former leukemia patient, you cannot donate tissues to other patients.

PART FIVE

Side Effects and Complications of Treatment

Will I need blood transfusions?

Are blood transfusions safe?

What side effects might a patient experience with chemotherapy?

More . . .

50. Will I need blood transfusions?

As you are being treated for leukemia, you might need to have **blood transfusions** as a consequence of the chemotherapy or because the disease itself has led to significant anemia or thrombocytopenia (low platelet count). Blood transfusions replenish red blood cells in the bloodstream when your own bone marrow is unable to do so. A threshold level of blood hematocrit or hemoglobin is selected by most physicians or hospitals for the use of blood transfusions to be considered (see Question 16). Because fatigue and shortness of breath are common symptoms of anemia, a blood transfusion will likely make you feel better almost immediately. Once it is determined that blood is needed, a unit of blood generally takes about 60 minutes to infuse into you. Generally, two units of blood are ordered, but occasionally, a physician will order only one unit to be infused.

Blood transfusion

Replenishment of red blood cells in the bloodstream when one's own bone marrow is unable to do so.

Platelet transfusions might be given if your platelet count reaches a critical level, as determined by your physician. Prophylactic platelet transfusions help prevent serious bleeding, a problem that can be life threatening if your platelet count is very low. If you have acute leukemia, you will likely need to undergo platelet transfusions during the intense phase of your treatment, and if you have chronic leukemia, you might need platelet transfusions in the later stages of disease.

Platelet transfusion

Procedure used in cancer patients to prevent or control bleeding when the number of platelets have decreased.

51. Are blood transfusions safe?

The simple answer to this question is, "yes." Screening for blood donors is very rigorous in order to exclude the transmission of infectious agents. Patients with high-risk behaviors, such as intravenous drug use or unprotected sex, are not allowed to donate blood under any circumstances. All donor units are screened for human immunodeficiency virus (HIV) and hepatitis B and C viruses. With this kind of testing, the risk of acquiring the hepatitis C virus is less than 1 in 100,000 units, the risk of acquiring hepatitis B virus is less than 1 in

63,000 units, and the risk of acquiring HIV is less than 1 in 750,000 units.

There are other, noninfectious risks of blood transfusion, including sudden destruction of the transfused red cells or even late destruction of the transfused red cells. This can give rise to serious complications, including kidney failure. However, these are very rare, and the benefit of transfusion far outweighs this small risk. Some patients also have a slight fever after a blood transfusion, which can be treated with acetaminophen (Tylenol).

Circulatory overload can occur occasionally in somebody with underlying congestive heart failure, but slow administration and perhaps the use of a diuretic medication can prevent this. Platelet transfusions carry the same infectious risks as blood transfusions, but they are equally well screened for infectious agents. Reaction to platelets sometimes occurs, consisting of fevers and chills. This, too, can be treated with medications like acetaminophen. The decision to give a blood or platelet transfusion is taken very seriously by a physician. When the decision is made to transfuse blood or platelets, the physician has determined that the benefits to the patient far outweigh any risks.

Blood products to be transfused into patients with leukemia are filtered to remove white blood cells in order to decrease potential immunization to white blood cell antigens that can lead to the development of autoantibodies; these auto-antibodies could, in turn, lead to destruction of platelets. In addition, blood and platelet units are treated with radiation to destroy white blood cells that might attack the patient (causing graft-versus-host disease; see Questions 62–64) while he or she is immunosuppressed by chemotherapy. Filtration and irradiation have made blood cell transfusions much safer, allowing the lifesaving nature of these treatments to be employed widely for leukemia.

52. What side effects might a patient experience with chemotherapy?

The **side effects** that are most common with leukemia patients include stomach upset up to the level of nausea and vomiting, mucositis (sore mouth), osteoporosis (thin bones), muscle weakness, severe energy depletion, reduced mental awareness, loss of appetite, blurred vision, loss of sexual desire, and headaches. The immediate effects of chemotherapy, such as nausea and vomiting, can be very well controlled with anti-nausea medications, and **analgesics** are available to handle the worst of the pain. The worst side effect of chemotherapy is the reduction in blood counts, leading to anemia, low platelet count, and low white blood cell count. Until chemotherapy or biologic therapy that can target only the leukemia cells exists, this side effect is unavoidable. **Mucositis** occurs when the lining of the inside of the mouth breaks down, making even swallowing painful. Liquid morphine is often prescribed for a short period so that patients can get adequate nourishment without experiencing the pain of mucositis. As the white counts continue to recover, this condition gradually abates.

All drugs are filtered through the body by the kidneys or are metabolized (broken down) by the liver. It is very important when someone is taking these treatments that he or she constantly flushes his or her body with fluids. When patients are in the hospital, they are usually given an intravenous infusion of a saline solution for that purpose. When they leave the hospital, they will be instructed to drink plenty of fluids. This could continue until their drug therapy is discontinued and kidney functions return to normal. Patients should have no alcoholic beverages until all medications are discontinued because alcohol inhibits the bone marrow, thus slowing down the recovery from chemotherapy. Alcohol can also injure the liver.

Drugs used to treat acute leukemia affect rapidly dividing cells. Unfortunately, hair follicles fall into that category. Therefore, it is fairly universal that patients with acute leukemia will lose their hair (**alopecia**) during chemotherapy. This means all hair. However, the hair will grow back. The loss of hair lasts for about 4–6 weeks, beginning about 7–14 days after the start of treatment. In some cases, the regrown hair will be slightly different in color and texture. That is only temporary, and the hair eventually will return to normal (see Question 60).

53. Will I lose weight after chemotherapy?

Typically, you will lose weight during treatment. When you are in the hospital, it will be harder to consume an adequate number of calories because of the nature of cafeteria-style food and the lack of appetite induced by chemotherapy. However, it is important to maintain your nourishment. Your physician and dietitian might agree that you may have food that meets their standards, but that would also taste good, brought in from home. You might find that much of the time, you have difficulty tolerating food due to mucositis and nausea. You might also notice a change in the way certain foods taste. This is only temporary, and taste returns to normal after the medications are discontinued.

54. Are there any proven herbal remedies that reduce side effects or that have therapeutic effects?

There is great interest in **alternative medicine** (i.e., nontraditional medical supplements or techniques) in the United States. Modern antinausea drugs (called **antiemetics**), blood cell growth factors, and antibiotics are doing a great job in limiting side effects already. In addition, despite claims that mushroom extracts and other so-called natural remedies have therapeutic effects in leukemia and other cancers, there is no credible evidence to back up these assertions. In fact, some products can even be harmful. The patient should beware of information from the Internet and nonscientific publications that could give the impression that the cure for leukemia is somehow being kept secret. Patients should not consider information regarding alternative medicines or treatments found

Alopecia
Hair loss.

Alternative medicine
Nontraditional medical supplements or techniques.

Antiemetic
Medicine that prevents or relieves nausea and vomiting, used during and sometimes after chemotherapy.

Side Effects and Complications of Treatment

in print or Internet advertisements to be credible and unbiased. The FDA must approve all medicines used in the United States, and investigational medicines must have FDA clearance for studies of their safety and efficacy. Currently, however, the FDA does not regulate dietary supplements, which is why some outrageous claims are allowed to go unchallenged. Patients should be sure to discuss any questions they have about alternative medicines with their doctor. The doctor should be able to determine the validity of the claims and ensure that patients are receiving the best possible medicines and treatments. Patients should not resort to unproven methods of treatment. Those who are not convinced can seek a second opinion.

55. Do I need to be in the hospital to receive treatment?

Some leukemia treatments can easily be given in an outpatient setting. For example, oral drug therapy with imatinib mesylate for CML is entirely an outpatient treatment. On the other hand, the treatment of acute leukemia with combination chemotherapy usually is administered intravenously and sometimes by long infusion and requires hospitalization. Patients with acute leukema (AML, ALL) are usually kept in the hospital after their initial chemotherapy until their blood counts recover. Modern practice usually involves discharging the patient after each subsequent cycle of chemotherapy has been administered. Readmission to the hospital might be necessary for treatment of complications, such as infection or bleeding. The most common reason for readmission to the hospital is the treatment of systemic infection, the signs of which are usually fever and chills, fatigue, and a generally poor feeling (known as **malaise**).

Malaise

A condition marked by fatigue and overall poor feeling.

56. What types of infections do I need to be concerned about?

There are many infections that complicate treatment of leukemia or that are increased in frequency because of the leukemia itself. Patients with CML do not have a particularly high incidence of infection. Patients with CLL, on the other hand, do have a higher incidence of bacterial infections. If you have CLL and are receiving drug treatment, you would be at risk for pneumonia or other upper respiratory infection at a rate higher than the normal population.

Patients with acute leukemias are the most vulnerable to infections, and the risk depends on many factors, such as the level of neutrophils in the blood, how recently chemotherapy was administered, and host factors, such as age and general medical condition. Bacterial infections are most common, followed by viral infections, followed by fungal infections. Fever is usually the first sign of infection that should be called to your doctor's attention. Of course, patients with leukemia can also get the common cold, upper respiratory infections, and the flu. It could be difficult to differentiate some conditions from a more serious bloodstream infection by a bacterium during neutropenia. Your doctor will schedule regular blood tests and follow-up visits to ensure your overall health. However, it is your responsibility to take these tests in a timely manner. Your doctor should be told of any new symptoms that are noticed, particularly when you are undergoing treatment, or if you are neutropenic.

57. Are all complications treatable?

The treatment of leukemia involves the use of strong cytotoxic drugs that do not always differentiate normal from malignant cells (see Question 20). Those complications are reversible or treatable in that the symptoms can be managed. Many cytotoxic drugs cause nausea and vomiting, but routine use of very strong antinausea drugs has reduced the severity of this problem. Infections are certainly treatable. However, some patients do develop overwhelming infections that do not respond adequately to therapy, so although the infections are treatable, the treatment is not always successful. The treatment of childhood leukemia can result in some cognitive (thought) impairment and possibly some slowness in growth and development.

The alopecia that occurs in most patients who undergo chemotherapy is temporary (see Question 60).

58. Will I need to wear a mask? Will I be in isolation?

Infections that are commonly encountered are caused by microorganisms that already have colonized your body. Therefore, measures taken to reduce exposure to organisms carried by others are only part of the scenario. If you are going to receive chemotherapy for acute leukemia in the hospital, you will probably have a single room that is considered clean and safe from airborne organisms. You will probably not wear a mask in your room, but if you leave the unit you might be asked to wear a mask to minimize exposure to infections carried by others. However, masks themselves do little to prevent the spread of infection. Correct and frequent hand washing should be emphasized, and anyone who visits you and enters your room must wash correctly. Wash stations are located outside of most patient hospital rooms. Patients might need to frequently remind even hospital staff to wash before entering or performing procedures. You will not be isolated from visitors, but reasonable limitations on large numbers of visitors and of visitors with any signs of infection are recommended. Children who recently have been immunized with live viruses (e.g., polio) should be avoided.

You will not be isolated from visitors, but reasonable limitations on large numbers of visitors and of visitors with any signs of infection are recommended.

59. Will I be able to eat regular foods?

If you are being treated for one of the chronic leukemias, most likely you can eat whatever you desire. On the other hand, if you are under treatment for acute leukemia, you will have periods of low white blood cell counts because of both the disease and its treatment. During this time, you will need to be on a neutropenic diet, that is, a diet that does not contain foods that might transmit infectious agents, such as bacteria, fungi, and parasites (see Question 15). This means you should not eat certain fresh fruits and vegetables or sushi and other raw meats. Once your blood counts have recovered, you will be able to eat your regular foods again. As with any person, it makes sense to eat a balanced diet complete with adequate fiber. If you are suffering from any lingering nausea or symptoms of indigestion, you might wish to consult a dietitian who has previous experience with leukemia or lymphoma patients. Avoiding spicy, fatty, or acidic foods is generally a good idea.

The taste buds are affected by chemotherapy. Therefore, for some weeks to months, food might not taste the same. However, normal taste sensations should recover with time.

60. How long before my hair grows back?

Depending on the particular chemotherapy agents that you are given, regrowth of your hair should begin several weeks after the last chemotherapy administration. It will take several months for your hair to grow out fully. Notably, the color and texture of your hair could change on its return. Unfortunately, no remedy for hair loss with certain chemotherapy drugs has been found. Some patients cut their hair short before starting treatment to minimize the effect of the hair loss and to create an interesting new look.

Women are generally comfortable with wigs, and some like scarves or other homemade headgear. Men often get various hats to help mask the baldness. Although some people make a fashion statement and choose to shave their heads, for others, the loss of hair is a daily visual reminder that they are undergoing cancer treatment. Because patients are in control of very little during this process, presenting an attractive exterior to those around them empowers these patients and enhances their self-esteem at a difficult time in their lives. Often, patients in the hospital bring several soft caps that can be worn to sleep in, which make them feel more presentable to the various caretakers, nurses, and visitors with whom they come in contact.

61. What complications can I expect from total body irradiation (TBI)?

Total body irradiation (TBI) is associated with some nausea and vomiting during its administration. Like any therapy that will have effects on the bone marrow, it reduces blood counts and causes immunosuppression. Late side effects of TBI include the development of cataracts, hypothyroidism, joint necrosis, and possibly an increased incidence of secondary cancers, such as skin cancers and brain cancer. However, secondary cancers as complications of TBI are rare. Despite these complications, TBI is an important ingredient of the preparative regimen for allogeneic transplantation for acute and chronic myeloid leukemia.

62. What is graft–versus–host (GVHD) disease, and how is it related to BMT?

Graft-versus-host disease

A condition in which the lymphocytes from a donor's stem cells recognize certain antigens on the recipient (patient) as foreign.

Graft-versus-host disease (GVHD) is a complication of allogeneic stem cell transplantation in which the lymphocytes from the donor's stem cells recognize certain antigens in the recipient (patient) as foreign. Thus, the lymphocytes mount a reaction against the tissues of the patient, causing GVHD. The organs particularly affected are the skin, the liver, and the gastrointestinal tract.

63. What are the consequences of GVHD?

Graft-versus-leukemia effect

Occurs when the donor's lymphocytes attack the patient's leukemia cells directly and help in the eradication of the leukemia.

GVHD manifestations can range from mild to severe. Mild GVHD could consist only of a minor skin rash that responds to steroid therapy. This mild reaction actually is generally associated with a better outcome because there is some evidence that GVHD correlates with a **graft-versus-leukemia effect**. Graft-versus-leukemia effect means that the donor's lymphocytes attack the patient's leukemia cells directly and help in the eradication of the leukemia.

However, if GVHD is quite severe, more aggressive medical therapy must be initiated, which can lead to more complications. Moreover, aggressive forms of GVHD might not respond well to therapy and might eventually actually lead to death. If a physician recommends that a patient has aggressive therapy to combat GVHD, the patient should discuss the ramifications and duration of this therapy so that he or she understands its consequences.

64. What are the differences between acute and chronic GVHD?

Acute GVHD is defined as GVHD that develops in the first 100 days after transplantation. The organs involved, including the skin, liver, and gastrointestinal tract, are primarily affected, leading to skin rash, jaundice, and diarrhea. Chronic GVHD is more subtle and affects different organs. For example, the eyes or the mouth might become dry, there might be a rash inside the mouth, the skin might develop a thickening and tightening, and there might be chronic liver dysfunction.

65. What is CMV?

CMV stands for **cytomegalovirus**. This virus is similar to the herpes virus and can cause pneumonia, hepatitis, and gastrointestinal illness. CMV is a relatively common virus, and most people have already been exposed to it. However, it can reactivate during immunosuppression and lead to disease in immunocompromised patients. A blood test can detect early initiation of CMV reactivation. If the reactivation is detected, preemptive drug therapy with a drug called ganciclovir (Cytovene, Vitrasert) can be initiated. Alternatively, patients may be treated with ganciclovir prophylactically (preventively), irrespective of the results of the blood test.

Cytomegalovirus

A virus similar to herpes virus, which can cause pneumonia, hepatitis, and gastrointestinal illness.

66. Can I get the stem cell donor's allergies?

This has been described as a rare event after transplantation. It is not considered to be a major factor in choosing a donor because usually there is only one suitable donor, and the benefit of the therapeutic effect of the transplantation far outweighs any plausible risk of contracting an allergy.

67. What are other complications of stem cell transplantation?

As with chemotherapy in general for leukemia, the main complications of high-dose chemotherapy used in stem cell transplantation are infection, bleeding, and isolated toxicity to organs such as the liver, heart, lungs, or kidneys (rare). Organ toxicity is the state in which the organ ceases to function or functions ineffectively. Heart failure can occur rarely. Lung fibrosis and hypersensitivity reactions can occur after certain drugs are used in the transplantation process. The liver could develop a condition known as **venoocclusive disease** that can lead to liver failure in some patients. In some patients who receive the drug cyclophosphamide (Cytoxan), there can be bleeding from the bladder wall, leading to bloody urine for a period of days to weeks. There can be skin changes, such as darkened patches of skin known as **hyperpigmentation**. There can be changes in the fingernails and toenails, such as nail dropout or splintering.

Venoocclusive disease

A sometimes fatal condition that can lead to liver failure; requires rapid medical intervention.

Hyperpigmentation

Darkened patches of skin.

68. Will I lose my sexual desire after stem cell transplantation?

Many leukemia patients lose their sexual desire during the diagnosis process and after their diagnosis and/or during treatment. The uncertainty of the future is difficult for most couples to put aside. When one partner is facing such a health challenge, the focus changes in the relationship to survival and how best to accomplish it.

During active treatment, your body will need all of its energy to fight the side effects. Any particular organ damage or dysfunction, such as kidney failure, will further play a role in how long the recovery process will take. Some medications will also inhibit your physical ability to have sexual activity. Over time, measured in weeks to months, as you recover from therapy, your sexual desire and your ability to perform will improve and should return to your normal pattern.

PART SIX

Treatment Facilities and Healthcare Providers

How do I know that my doctor is providing the right treatment?

Is there a difference between an attending doctor and a fellow?

Do all hospitals perform all treatments?

More . . .

69. How do I know my doctor is providing the right treatment?

The first thing about being a good patient is that you need to be your own best advocate. The relationship you have with your doctor is like any other relationship. You must feel comfortable openly communicating with your doctor and ensuring that each of you are meeting each other's expectations. Read, read, and read more. Actively research your condition to ensure that you are aware of what your treatment options are. This will give you the tools to ensure you ask your doctor the right questions about your condition. While doctors are not always right, they do have more resources available to them to research any concerns or questions you might have. This will also allow you to better understand what is happening in your body and ensure you can explain your symptoms. Talk with others with leukemia, do research on the Internet, and confer with several doctors other than your own hematologist/oncologist about any issues that concern you. You have the final say about what your treatment options are. You are almost always free to decline any procedure and leave any facility at any time. Of course, you do this at your own risk. With the ever-changing medical arena and the increasing demands on our medical system, it becomes more and more important that you are aware of any and all treatment options available. Make sure to ask your doctor plenty of questions until you get a firm understanding of what is happening to you. The physicians who are licensed in this nation are the world's best trained and most dedicated, and most can do incredible things with their skills, knowledge, and dedication. Although patients like to think that their doctors are the best, no doctor is perfect. The medical community might never fully understand how the entire human body functions. That is why they call it practicing medicine. If you feel that your treatment is not progressing as well as you would like, talk to your doctor about other treatments or facilities that might better accommodate you. As a patient, you must have confidence in nurses and technicians, as well as physicians, **caregivers**, and all others who care for you. Make sure you are as well informed as they are to ensure your treatment progresses. Time is not always on your side.

Caregiver

Acts for the benefit of a patient at the time of serious illness or disease, on the patient's behalf, and assists the patient in making decisions and choices.

During your treatment for leukemia, many issues arise. No answer should be accepted unless you understand it and are aware of its repercussions. A physician's time can be very limited because of the increased caseload that most carry. All questions or concerns should be answered on a daily basis while the doctor is examining you, whether you are hospitalized or under care in the outpatient setting.

There are great doctors, good doctors, and not-so-good doctors. You should have confidence in your doctor's abilities. Assess his qualifications and ensure they are to your standards. One gauge for determining whether you have a great doctor is whether he or she always spends the appropriate amount of time to explain all issues in layman's terms to you and your caregiver. The doctor should always ask this question before leaving, "Do you have any further questions?"

You should always strive to acquire the best medical care available—the choice of physician can be the most important factor in a quick and successful return to good health. Second opinions are often recommended, especially if the clinical situation is not straightforward, or if the proposed treatment is not standard.

70. Is there a difference between an attending doctor and a fellow?

Those who are being treated in a hospital setting will be exposed to many different professionals. The medical team will be led by an **attending physician**. This term applies to a fully licensed and board-certified/eligible physician who is on the faculty of the institution or the medical staff. A **fellow** is a licensed physician who is still in training. A fellow in hematology/oncology will have already completed 3 years of internal medicine training and likely will have taken boards in that discipline already. The certification agency is referred to as the American Board of Internal Medicine. At the completion of 2–3 years of hematology/oncology training, the fellow is then eligible to sit for the hematology and oncology boards, also

Attending physician

A fully licensed and board-certified/ eligible physician who is on the faculty of the institution or the medical staff.

Fellow

A licensed physician who is still in training.

administered by the American Board of Internal Medicine. Therefore, a fellow is a highly trained individual already, who is now honing his or her skills in the more specific discipline of hematology/oncology.

Patients might also encounter medical residents, depending on the institution. Medical residents and interns are physicians who have received their medical degree from a certified medical school. They are in training in internal medicine, which is the parent discipline for hematology/oncology. Patients might also encounter medical students who are in their third or fourth year of medical school. Medical students will be under close supervision by licensed and certified physicians.

71. Do all hospitals perform all treatments?

With technology advancing daily, not all hospitals are capable of performing the most advanced tests and procedures that a leukemia patient might need. In addition, small community hospitals are not staffed for and oriented to the level of intensity of care that a leukemia patient requires. For this reason, it is recommended that chemotherapy for leukemia be delivered in a hospital that is prepared for the complications that can arise. This might or might not be an academic health center or a large community hospital with experienced staff. In our estimation, the hospital should have a track record of delivering such treatments to at least 20 patients per year. Hospitals affiliated with major cancer centers are most likely to be oriented to the treatment of leukemia patients. The National Cancer Institute (NCI), a branch of the National Institutes of Health, recognizes certain institutions as either clinical or comprehensive cancer centers through a peer-reviewed mechanism that ensures quality. Patients are more likely to receive up-to-date care and access to innovative clinical trials at institutions that have met the high standards of the National Cancer Institute. However, many non-National Cancer Institute–designated cancer centers, hospitals, and private clinics offer excellent services, too. Patients should research

Hospitals affiliated with major cancer centers are most likely to be oriented to the treatment of leukemia patients.

the possible places of treatment in their area. All of the hospitals have details about the doctors available there and what their medical backgrounds are. If a better hospital is available in or near a patient's home but there are financial or physical transportation difficulties, several nonprofit agencies offer assistance in getting patients to the facility.

If a patient's leukemia is not responding to the **standard protocol** or if the treatment is causing other medical issues, a variety of clinical trials might be available (see Question 29). Hospitals and cancer centers each have access to their own clinical trials. Not all treatment options are available at all hospitals. If a hematologist/oncologist recommends or informs a patient of studies that are available, the patient should be sure to investigate all options available. It is ultimately the patient's responsibility to make an informed decision about his or her treatment. A doctor might inform patients only of clinical trials that are available at his or her hospital and might not be aware of all that is available. The Internet can be a very useful tool in locating information in this area, and the National Cancer Institute has a web page listing current, NCI-approved clinical trials. See Question 100 and the Appendix for some of the most common and useful web sites.

Standard protocol

Treatment generally recognized by the medical community as the standard of care.

72. Is there an agency with survival statistics for different treatments and BMTs?

The best source of information for leukemia treatments, including bone marrow transplantation, are the Leukemia & Lymphoma Society of America, the National Marrow Donor Program (NMDP), the Multiple Myeloma Association, the Myelodysplastic Foundation, the International Bone Marrow Transplant Registry (IBMTR), and the American Society of Bone Marrow Transplantation. The American Society of Hematology and the American Society of Clinical Oncology (ASCO) have useful information, as does the American Cancer Society (ACS). Contact information for these organizations can be found in the Appendix.

73. How important is the nurse's role in my overall care and survival?

Nurses are in the third most important category of caregivers in your life as a patient being treated for leukemia. Only your oncologist and caregiver are more essential. Nurses perform their duties and care as instructed by the physician.

The nursing shortage in this country is growing, and there are not enough qualified nursing schools to educate the number of students that are needed. Hospitals have had to lower the standard of care by using technicians for patient care. With leukemia patients, this is of particular concern, because the care they need is very critical. Doctors instruct by writing or speaking orders, but the nurses carry out the elements of care. Aides or medical assistants have only 2 years of medical training, which is much different than a 4-year nursing degree. These personnel are very helpful in your care, but they require supervision.

In addition to technicians, many nursing shifts are now being staffed temporarily by licensed vocational nurses (LVNs) instead of registered nurses (RNs) due to the shortage. Nurses brought in on a temporary basis are called traveling nurses. They contract with a medical facility for a short period (usually about 13 weeks). Although they are qualified professionals, most are not familiar enough with the facility and the staff to be able to offer the best possible care.

You should talk to your nurse and ask questions. It is your right as a patient to advise the charge nurse if you feel that you have an incompetent or inattentive nurse, and if this is the case, you should ask for that nurse to be replaced by another. If the problem is not resolved, the director of nursing and the attending physician should be notified. Although the nurse's position is very demanding, the margin for error is very limited and should not be tested. Remember that your health is at stake.

It is also important to have your caregiver (see Questions 74–82) with you when all blood products are given to ensure accurate observation and documentation. Most states require that two nurses check all data with you before blood is infused. You will need to answer several questions, including date of birth and Social Security number, for verification to ensure you are given the proper treatment.

74. What are the functions of a caregiver?

Caregivers are very important to the outcome of a serious illness or disease. Each is part cheerleader, administrator, counselor, secretary, nurse, and chauffeur. The patient, at times, might be totally dependent on others to stay alive.

The caregiver steps in for the benefit of another at the time of serious illness or disease. The patient might be mentally fatigued by what seems like a relentless amount of medical advice and alternatives to treatment or might be physically challenged by the treatment itself. It is the role of the caregiver to not only be there for emotional support but also to help the patient decipher all of the information given, so that the patient is able to make the best choice. The caregiver should have a willing spirit to go the distance when needed. A caregiver can be a spouse, family member, friend, or professional caregiver.

The stress and the emotional and physical limitations of losing your health to leukemia are most difficult. You are faced with a tremendous number of critical decisions that could and will affect the chances of your survival. You need a competent support structure of caregivers who are able to discuss issues as they arise and make decisions as necessary. Medications, lab tests, and procedures should all be documented—depending on the medical staff to always have all your details at their fingertips is unrealistic.

75. What should you expect from the caregiver/patient relationship?

The most important part of the caregiver/patient relation-ship is a mutual respect for one another that allows you to trust the person who is responsible for your well-being. You and your caregiver will spend an incredible amount of time together and will forge a relationship like no other. Leukemia is often an emotional roller coaster for both the patient and the caregiver. Thus, the caregiver will need to learn as much as possible about your disease or illness and become familiar with the plan for medical care. The caregiver should always be on alert to your emotional status, because a positive attitude is essential for your successful recovery. Your caregiver must be honest, forthcoming with information, kind, caring, and loving. He or she must be a good listener and a friend, and most importantly, must have patience.

76. How important is the caregiver?

It is very difficult to go through aggressive treatment for leu-kemia, particularly during periods of intense chemotherapy. Doing this alone would be very difficult for anyone. There-fore, the caregiver is most important for helping patients go through the acute phases of treatment. In addition to help-ing with basic needs, including eating, personal hygiene, and elimination, the caregiver also is extremely important for giving emotional support. Caregivers can provide an outlet for patients and be someone they can always talk to. Some caregivers have gone through this process with other patients and have their own experiences and insights to offer. They can also provide advice to the patient's family.

77. Should the caregiver keep a patient chart?

During chemotherapy and radiation treatments, a patient's physical and emotional well-being are taxed severely. Doctors present procedures that require decisions coupled with statis-tics that can often determine a patient's survival. The patient is constantly dealing with numbers—for blood counts, drug side effects, urination and stool quantities, and all other medical issues. This requires someone, in addition to the medical staff, to keep accurate records. Doctors are very busy and go on rounds to see patients every day, asking many questions. If the caregiver can become an expert on the patient and his or her condition and give answers quickly and accurately, the medical staff might be more forthcoming with patient information. This means that the patient and the caregiver will have a better understanding of the current medical conditions.

Keeping a detailed record of lab values and treatments is useful also in navigating the complexity of the healthcare system. Because a patient might be under the care of more than one doctor, any one doctor, hospital, or clinic might not have access to some or all of the patient's medical records. An organized summary of events, kept in a notebook, can be very useful during an office or hospital visit.

Many treatment facilities have electronic medical records systems that can be accessed online by the doctor, patient, and potentially a delegate. It is a good method to keep track of your prescriptions, appointments, and test results. Don't hesitate to ask your doctor about getting access or for a hard copy of your lab results and visit information even if you have switched to a different physician.

The caregiver and the family need to keep communication with the patient in the most positive and loving manner possible. This is most important in successfully surviving the most difficult time of life. Without a great caregiver, chances of a successful outcome are greatly reduced. Patients without family should have trusted and willing friends fill this role.

78. Are caregivers needed in the hospital?

Yes, most definitely. The caregiver is the **patient's advocate**. The patient must focus on getting well and not be sidetracked

Patient advocate

An individual who serves the needs of the patient, who may be empowered to act on his or her behalf.

on issues that are best left up to others. The caregiver should make decisions on when best to step in if critical medical care is not being performed at the highest level.

While someone is in the hospital, it is also important to have the caregiver available most of the time. The medical staff cannot provide support to patients as well as the family does. When problems arise, it is very helpful for the patient to have the support of loved ones. Having someone to talk with and discuss the current issues with is a huge benefit.

Caregivers should never leave the patient unattended for any length of time. There must be someone with them throughout their stay to watch, listen, record, and ask questions about what is going on. Basically, the caregiver is a monitor to ensure that everything that is supposed to occur actually happens. If there is a problem, it should be reported; this is not a time to be silent for fear of hurting someone's feelings.

Hospitalizations can be long and arduous, filled with long days and nights. The caregiver should get rest when possible and take breaks when others come to visit. The conversations should be kept light and positive. Patients are sometimes unable to see past the walls in the room, so they can easily become depressed, bored, and filled with anxiety. Music is often therapeutic and can be encouraged.

The food prepared in the hospital is often quite bland and might not appeal to patients whose taste buds have been altered due to the therapy being given. With the approval and knowledge of the physician and dietitian, the caregiver may either supplement or fully attend to the patient's wishes for the nourishment desired. It is often a real treat to have some special food items brought in. This must be done cautiously because leukemia patients are immunosuppressed and could become very ill or even die if they ingest food that their systems cannot handle. The caregiver should always get permission before bringing food that is prepared out of the hospital.

79. Do caregivers get any training?

Many medical institutions have classes and groups in caregiving. After treatment and in-home care, the caregiver needs to administer medications and communicate with the hospital staff on a regular basis. Knowing what to do and how to do it is essential to accelerate the healing process. The patient's main goals should be to follow all the doctor's orders and to get discharged home as soon as medically possible. The caregiver is essential in helping to achieve these goals.

80. Can and should family members be caregivers?

Your family is most important, with each member filling different needs. Caregiving can be more demanding for the provider than for the patient because the patient is often medicated. The love and support from family members is often the single most important reason that patients have for doing their very best to survive during the most difficult of times. Fighting leukemia and going through the regimens of treatments is not for the faint of heart—it is tough. The thought of not seeing your family any longer produces a great motivation. The best medication is unable to create such a response. Determining whether a family member should be a caregiver should be discussed in great length with the physician, the family member, and the patient. The family member must understand what is required and expected of him or her if he or she becomes a caregiver. Being a caregiver is very difficult and time consuming. If a family member is too distant from the situation, he or she might not be the best caregiver for the patient. If an experienced caregiver can offer better care, it is best to choose that caregiver over a family member.

Fighting leukemia and going through the regimens of treatments is not for the faint of heart—it is tough.

81. How involved should family members be with the patient?

Family members should be involved with the patient in order to provide emotional support. However, it is also important for family members to respect the privacy and the need for rest and solitude that the patient needs from time to time. Family members can be helpful in being the patient's advocate to the healthcare system. During the acute phases of treatment, the patient might not be in the position to ask questions or might feel reticent about complaining. It is important for the family to be aware of what is going on with the patient and to make sure that symptoms are brought to the attention of the patient's doctor.

Many times family members feel uncomfortable talking about difficult issues. Family members should not hesitate to talk to the patient. A warm, caring voice is always welcome. Relatives who are not close should call the patient's immediate family and ask if it would be appropriate to contact the patient directly. A patient remembers who did and didn't call during treatment. Many families grow closer during these times, but many also drift apart. Staying in touch with the patient is the best way relatives can show that they care.

82. What is the impact of family as caregivers?

The positive impact that the family brings to a patient is enormous. The love and support from family are often the single biggest reason patients strive to do their best during the most difficult times. Each family member can fill different needs and accomplish different tasks. It helps to have a different face with a new conversation to help keep the mood uplifting and fresh. No medications can mirror a response as great as the love of a family member or close friend.

83. Are all medical facilities the same?

Many patients feel that the larger the medical facility is, the better it must be. Sometimes, this is the case, but assumptions should not be made when the stakes are so high. Patients should always be curious about the qualifications of a facility and its physicians and staff. Before any treatment is performed, patients should visit the center and interview the physicians responsible for the care that their illness requires. Many medical centers have background information about the physicians, including where they studied and their experiences with different types of leukemia and lymphoma. With medical care, ignorance is not bliss. The patient must become as knowledgeable as possible in a short period of time. Talking to experts in the care and treatment of the disease is essential in gaining that knowledge.

Although most large cancer centers receive the greatest portion of government and private funding, the performance of smaller institutions should not be overlooked. Many excellent physicians prefer to practice in smaller centers where the bureaucracy is less intrusive and thus more time can be dedicated to the patients.

One criterion that can be used in evaluating the best possible facility is whether the institution has substantial experience in treating all types of leukemia. This assurance means that the doctors and all the support staff are equally experienced and are likely to be familiar with a particular type of leukemia. Because a patient will have significant communication with his or her physician and the physician's staff, the physician and staff should be easily accessible.

Before a patient makes the final decision, he or she should talk with some of the nurses and determine the level of care available at the facility. Common sense can be as good as facts and figures. Patients must feel comfortable that they will receive the best care possible to encourage the necessary level of trust.

84. How can the patient show his or her appreciation toward the medical staff?

The medical staff is like any other dedicated group of people. Professional personnel like to be shown respect and appreciation. These professionals involved in patient care have a very demanding job. Tokens of gratitude are well advised and can make a difference in the attitude that a patient receives. As with any relationship, one receives what one puts into it. These medical support members must care for people when they are, many times, at their worst. With this type of environment, an act of kindness goes a long way.

A good way to show appreciation is to make a monetary donation to the facility. A donation can be targeted to a specific program or for the benefit of an individual's research program. The availability of research funding from the federal government has decreased. Philanthropic support of research is more important than ever, especially since there are so many new ideas, new highly active treatments, and new technologies that need to be tested and validated in clinical studies. Charitable donations are very much appreciated. If you are interested in making a donation, ask your doctor or social worker for a contact with the proper professionals involved in gifting.

There are always new patients that are afflicted by leukemia and lymphoma. They do not know what to expect of their treatment. Some are scared and confused. Volunteering to meet with these patients even if just to relay experiences or listen to them is always helpful. A family member not afflicted with leukemia or lymphoma is also welcome to volunteer. They have their own experiences and points of view that might help these patients and their families understand and cope with the disease. Many cancer patients—not just those with leukemia—have to deal with the same problems. Volunteers shouldn't limit themselves to a particular kind of leukemia. It is also a great idea to volunteer at other local nonprofit organizations. Larger organizations have volunteer programs.

85. What is the employer's responsibility to its employees pertaining to leave of absence for treatment of leukemia?

An employee is entitled to 12 weeks of family leave of absence (Family Medical Leave Act, also known as FMLA). The employee's same job or a comparable position is guaranteed on his or her return during these 12 weeks. Also, the health insurance benefits are continued as if the employee was still working during this time period. In other words, if the employee was paying $200 per month for his or her health insurance coverage, and if the employee continues to pay the same amount to the employer, the benefits will continue through this period. In California and several other states, the employee can apply for state disability benefits so that additional income can be awarded while the employee is unable to work.

If the employee is unable to return to work after 12 weeks, the employer can terminate employment. In fact, most companies have a standard policy that is applied when the 12 weeks of FMLA are exhausted. At this point, the employee is removed from the payroll and the separation papers are completed. The employee is eligible by law to apply for continuation of health coverage (mandated by the Consolidated Omnibus Budget Reconciliation Act of 1985 [COBRA]). Under COBRA, the employer can charge the employee the full cost of the group healthcare plan plus a 2% administrative fee. In other words, if the employee has been paying $200 and the employer was paying the remainder of $300, the employee at this point would be responsible for $500 plus an additional 2%.

This healthcare continuation coverage is still under the employer's group plan. If payment from the employee is not received within 30 days of the date established by the employer each period, whether it is monthly or quarterly, the employer can cancel the health coverage at that time. It is advisable to send the funds by certified mail or in person and get documented receipts because this coverage is vital to a patient's continued care. In most cases, the COBRA coverage continues by law for 18 months. If another qualifying event (e.g., death of a covered spouse) occurs, then the coverage extends to 36 months. A disability provision could extend the 18-month COBRA period to total coverage of 29 months. Because these issues can get rather complicated, and the laws can and do change, a good source of up-to-date information is the local or state Chamber of Commerce. Consulting a social worker can help patients find alternate healthcare coverage solutions.

86. When all else fails, how do I prepare my family and myself for my death?

Too few people think ahead to what happens should cancer get the better of them. Even knowing that leukemia can be a fatal disease, most people with it prefer to concentrate instead on curing the cancer—an understandable attitude that is to be encouraged. As time passes and the cancer advances, however, there comes a point when cancer patients should start thinking about what they want to have happen should they lose the battle.

As difficult as it might be to contemplate your own death, doing so before the end is imminent can ease matters for you and your family if your leukemia follows that course. Everyone hopes such arrangements would not be necessary, but it is useful to work out those legal arrangements that might be required ahead of time (while you're still feeling relatively well). Then, with the details of your will, power of attorney designation, a do not resuscitate (DNR) order (see Question 87), funeral arrangements, and other practical matters out of the way, it is easier to focus on your health, knowing that these structures are in place. There are several steps you can take to accomplish this.

Work toward acceptance. Even after a long, difficult illness, it's very hard to accept that you're going to die within the next few months or weeks. Preparing yourself for death is a major emotional and spiritual undertaking, so get assistance from a minister, social worker, or psychologist. If you don't have a clergyman or counselor with whom you're comfortable, most cancer centers or oncology wards have a chaplain or counselor in residence. Take advantage of their services, or ask for a referral. Involve your family in some of these sessions, but use as many as you need just for yourself—if you can gain a sense of peace for yourself, it will help your family to cope with your death, too. Ironically, achieving this sort of peace and acceptance can help you to live longer than predicted; it's not unheard of people who are believed to have but a few months remaining to live many months, even years, after making their final arrangements for death.

You have a right to receive **palliative treatment**, a type of therapy that relieves symptoms, such as pain or fatigue, but does not alter the development of the disease. Its primary purpose is to improve the quality of your life.

Because many people find this time hard to think about and talk about, it's likely that you'll have to raise the issue with your family, friends, and healthcare team. Your loved ones might resist the discussion, but be persistent—or get help from a social worker, counselor, or clergy who can guide them through this painful conversation. It's important to talk about what you want to happen in the final phases of your illness. Discuss the organization of personal documents and where they are kept so that your family and friends know what your wishes and desires are. Lawyers, clergy, and counselors can also help you and your family in planning for end-of-life issues.

Decide on the best place for your care. People facing advanced cancer should choose the location of their care: in the home, in an outpatient setting or the doctor's office, in the hospital, or through a hospice. Although people can live with recurrent disease for a long time, at some point people with advanced disease experience a shift in which it becomes clear that they are dying. It might be best to discuss the decision of where you would like to be treated for advanced cancer before this point if you can. Hospice care focuses on improving the quality of life for the remainder of your life and can make the process of dying as comfortable and as pain free as possible. Hospice care can be given in the home, at the hospital, or in a hospice.

Palliative treatment

Therapy that relieves symptoms but does not alter the development of the disease. Its primary purpose is to improve the quality of life.

These are all personal choices based on your needs and available resources. Your healthcare team can discuss these options with you and help you get the care you need.

Make your wishes known. If cancer treatment becomes unbearable, you have the right to request that your doctors stop treatment. You even have the ability to describe in writing what kinds of treatment you will and will not accept from them, in case you should lose the ability to communicate your wishes directly. Legal documents called **advance directives**, including living wills, durable powers of attorney, **do not resuscitate (DNR) orders**, and healthcare proxies allow you to express your decisions regarding what you do and don't want to have done during your last weeks or months, in case you become unable to communicate effectively at that time. These are described in Question 87.

Advance directives

Legal documents spelling out how you want your treatment to proceed, including living wills, DNR orders, and durable power of attorney.

Do not resuscitate order

A medical order telling the medical staff at the hospital or facility that they should not act to revive you in the event that your heart or brain activity cease.

87. Are there legal steps I can take to make my wishes known in case I'm not able to speak for myself near the end?

You have the right to decide what treatment you will and will not accept near the end of your life, and you also have the right to designate an individual to speak for you—this is usually a member of your family, but it can be a friend or an attorney. You don't need an official document or form—you don't even need to have this document written by an attorney. All you really need to do is sign a letter in the presence of two or more witnesses (who should also sign and date the document). However, if the letter is notarized, it will carry more weight with a hospital board, if questions should arise.

Living will

Document outlining what care you want in the event that you become unable to communicate due to coma or heavy sedation.

Advance directives dictate how you want your treatment to proceed, including **living wills**, DNR orders, durable powers of attorney, and healthcare proxies. A living will simply outlines what care you want in the event that you become unable to communicate due to coma or heavy sedation. You're not locked into anything you write down. The document is nothing more than a legally valid guide for your family and physicians to know your thinking on how you should be cared for. If you change your mind about any of it, you can change the directives or even verbally countermand them to the physician treating you. Alternatively, you can limit the instructions to a do not resuscitate order (DNR) if you decide differently, telling the medical staff at the hospital that they should not act to revive you in the event your heart or respiratory activity (breathing) cease.

Even if you don't write it down, if you have certain ideas as to what kind of treatment you do and don't want, all you need to do is tell members of your family, particularly those acting as your principal caregivers. If they know your wishes, they can intervene on your behalf even without a written statement—although they might have to convince a judge that this is truly your wish, if the hospital should balk at their requests to withhold treatment. Your family will then be bolstered if you prepare, in advance, a **durable power of attorney** (which allows a specific family member to legally make all your decisions, personal and financial, for you in case you become incapacitated). Another document you can prepare is a **healthcare proxy**, which limits the decision-making power to only those decisions regarding your medical treatment.

If you don't have a will, one should be written as soon as possible, particularly if you have children. If you fail to do this, most states' laws arrange for your assets to go directly to your spouse and children in specific proportions. However, processing your estate can take considerably more time without a will, which can cause problems for your family if bank accounts, property, or savings are held solely in your name. Different circumstances might create other mitigating factors—prior marriages with or without children, common-law marriages, or other nontraditional relationships. In these instances, having a will clarifies your wishes and is a tremendous kindness

Durable power of attorney

Allows a specific family member to legally make all your decisions, personal and financial, for you in case you become incapacitated.

Healthcare proxy

Document that limits the decision-making power to only those decisions about your medical treatment.

to your loved ones. Some people also make advanced arrangements for their funerals, which can be particularly helpful to your family, because they won't be confronted with these details in the midst of grieving over your death. It might be difficult—there is no more stark confrontation with your impending mortality than arranging your own funeral. However, knowing that this detail has already been dealt with can also help bring a measure of acceptance and peace.

PART SEVEN

Living with Leukemia

How does someone know whether he or she is cured?

Will my child with leukemia grow up normally?

Do patients ever get back to normal?

More . . .

88. *How does someone know whether he or she is cured?*

Certain forms of leukemia are indeed curable. These include ALL, AML, and CML. Unfortunately, present treatments are generally not considered curative for CLL, although allogeneic bone marrow transplantation may cure some patients with this disease. For all forms of leukemia there is always a slight chance of relapse. Long-term follow-up of patients with acute leukemia and CML patients who have undergone allogeneic bone marrow transplantation have indicated that some patients never have a relapse. When sufficient follow-up has taken place over a number of years with no sign of leukemia, it can be concluded that the patient is, in fact, cured. The first step toward cure is the achievement of a complete remission (total absence of disease) after initial therapy. In some cases, this can be determined by examining the blood and bone marrow cells under a microscope to discover whether there are residual blasts. More refined techniques, such as molecular markers and chromosomal abnormalities, might be used as well to ensure that no hidden cells exist. There are certain prognostic features that predict with some certainty who is most likely to suffer a relapse; these are discussed in the section on cytogenetics (Question 18). In the initial phases of the remission, it is difficult to state with any certainty whether a given patient is cured, because it takes many follow-up visits to be sure that a cure really occurred. Thus, it is not easy for the physician to tell a patient that he or she is cured early after treatment. In the case of the acute types of leukemia, after initial chemotherapy is completed, if the patient remains in complete remission for several years, it becomes more likely that the patient is in fact cured. The 5-year survival numbers are often given when reporting outcomes of certain studies. Generally, if the patient survives 5 years after therapy, relapse is unlikely, but, unfortunately, not unheard of. Thus, the word "cure" must be taken with a grain of salt because occasionally a patient relapses 7, 8, or more years after treatment.

Nonetheless, when a patient has survived for a long period of time after treatment, although there is some possibility of relapse, it becomes less common, and most patients have no difficulty putting their illness behind them. The fact that relapses can occur just means that patients must continue to follow up with their doctors.

CML is curable by allogeneic bone marrow transplantation. When performed in the first chronic phase, especially early after diagnosis of CML, allogeneic bone marrow transplantation has a very high cure rate, and the relapse rate is very low. If the transplantation is performed at a later stage of the disease, such as after a relapse, there is a higher probability of relapse. The new treatment recently established for CML using the drugs known as tyrosine kinase inhibitors [e.g., imatinib mesylate (Gleevec)] produces remissions in a large percentage of patients. At present, it is unknown whether these remissions will result in cures.

89. Will my child with leukemia grow up normally?

The combination of chemotherapy and central nervous system radiation therapy involved in the treatment of ALL does have a cost in terms of growth and development and neurologic function later in life. These effects are variable and seem to be more common in younger children (less than 5 years of age), and possibly more in girls than in boys. Survivors of childhood ALL tend to have shorter height than their unaffected counterparts. There is also a higher incidence of cataracts and cardiac abnormalities. Gonadal function usually develops normally unless the patient has had prophylactic gonadal irradiation. Successfully treated children with ALL have gone on to bear normal children in adulthood. Secondary cancers, including brain tumors, acute myeloid leukemia, and rare carcinomas of the parotid and thyroid glands, are more common after treatment of ALL. Hopefully, new advances in treatment will allow less intense treatment or treatment with different agents that decrease some of the side effects of treating ALL.

90. Do patients ever get back to normal?

In contrast to childhood ALL, patients treated for adult forms of leukemia who are successfully induced into remission will eventually find that they feel well and normal again. The time it takes to achieve this goal varies between patients and is affected by age and other medical illnesses or disorders that the patient has. Lingering fatigue can plague a patient for several months or even a year, but it eventually improves, depending on the intensity of treatment that the patient achieved, any other illnesses he or she has, age, prior fitness, and many other individual factors. Patients treated for the chronic leukemias might find that they feel much better after treatment has started because they might have better blood counts and better control of side effects of the elevated white blood cell counts. Being treated with an agent like imatinib mesylate, for example, is not really associated with very many side effects at all.

91. Do patients with leukemia develop other forms of cancer?

As mentioned earlier, children treated for ALL have a higher incidence of secondary neoplasms (cancers that develop later). Patients with CLL have a higher incidence of colon cancer and certain skin cancers. Patients treated for AML tend not to have a higher incidence of other cancers, if they are cured of the AML. Patients with CML do not have an increased incidence of secondary cancers. CML can evolve into a more aggressive form of leukemia that behaves essentially like AML.

92. Will I be able to have children?

Chemotherapy and radiation therapy can cause sterility. However, many patients who have been treated as children for acute leukemia have been able to have children of their own.

If you are a young adult man, it would be advisable to collect sperm before chemotherapy or before bone marrow transplantation to ensure that you could later father a child through artificial insemination if you prove infertile. For women, it is possible to harvest and store ova (eggs), but the procedure is more invasive, more expensive, and might not be covered by insurance. In weighing the decision to collect sperm or harvest ova before treatment, bear in mind that fertility is still possible even after aggressive chemotherapy for adult leukemia. Nevertheless, many male and female patients do become sterile, and you must be prepared for this possibility. Each treatment can have a different risk level of infertility; it is important to discuss these concerns with a physician and significant other to determine the best course of action.

93. When can I go back to work?

The answer to this question depends on the type of treatment you have received. Again, chronic leukemias might not necessitate ever leaving work unless the leukemia has advanced to an acute form or you undergo stem cell transplantation. If you are treated for acute leukemia, you need to stop working for some or all of the time during treatment. After the treatment has been completed, you may resume work within a few weeks to months. If your blood counts are depressed or there is ongoing immunosuppression, common sense approaches to avoiding infections will be recommended, such as avoiding crowds and washing hands frequently.

94. What are the patient's physical limitations after a bone marrow transplantation?

After an autologous transplantation, a patient usually bounces back to normal within a few months—there should really be no physical limitations. After an allogeneic transplantation, there might be numerous ongoing concerns, including active GVHD or active immunosuppression. The patient's blood counts and overall status generally dictate physical limitations. Certainly, walking and activities of normal daily living would be expected to return to normal within a few months, but vigorous exercise or exertion might not be recommended for several months to a year after transplantation (see Question 95).

95. When can I start to exercise after transplantation? Does exercise play a role in my recovery?

Light exercise—that is, walking and passive muscle movement—is recommended even during a bone marrow transplantation or chemotherapy in general. After completion of treatment, you should try to resume activities including walking and light exercise. If you have not been involved in vigorous exercise, this is probably not the time to start. However, if you have previously been physically fit and very involved in exercise routines, it is not unreasonable to gradually reintroduce your previous activities, depending on your blood counts and other physical factors. If anemia has been corrected and if low platelet counts are not a problem, then there are no true limitations to physical activities.

The general rule for exercise is a 20-minute routine a minimum of 3 days a week. This could be a brisk walk and some weight-bearing exercises, and it can be done any time, if your blood counts and your physician permit it. Everything should be done in moderation. The body will not perform at peak levels while in treatment. This can be frustrating. The key is to keep a routine going, especially if you are restricted to a bed for much of the day. During your treatment in the hospital, your doctor will encourage you to walk the halls regularly. In the first weeks, this will be very difficult. Exercise is good for you physically and mentally to reduce anxiety and stress. Your caregiver should help you stay motivated. You should consider consulting a physical therapist to give you instruction and ideas if routine exercise has not been a part of your daily life previously.

96. *What is the chance of the leukemia coming back?*

This question must be answered in relation to each form of leukemia as well as each stage and subtype of leukemia. This question also assumes that a remission has been achieved. If a patient with AML achieves a complete remission, then there is roughly a 60% chance that the disease will come back. If a child with ALL achieves a complete remission, the chance of recurrence is about 20%. If an adult with ALL achieves complete remission, the chance of relapse is about 60%. Patients with CML are currently being treated with one of the new drugs, imatinib mesylate (Gleevec), dasatinib (Sprycel), or nilotinib (Tasigna). For patients that have a good response to one of these agents, relapse rates are very low. It may be necessary to continue taking one of these medications for life. At this time, it is uncertain what the relapse rate will be in those who do respond to the drug. Patients who are taken off of these medications experience a high rate of relapse. Increasing numbers of patients with CLL are achieving remission with emerging therapies. After bone marrow transplantations, the relapse rates are also variable, depending on the disease and when the transplantation was performed. For example, if the patient has AML and undergoes an autologous transplantation in first complete remission, the relapse rate is approximately 40%. If the patient undergoes an autologous transplantation in second complete remission, the relapse rate is 60%. If a patient with CML undergoes an allogeneic stem cell transplantation, the relapse rate is approximately 10% in chronic phase, 30% in accelerated phase, and 50% in blastic crisis. Thus, the overall complexity of the variables involved in the leukemia, its biology, the mode of treatment, and other factors all influence the relapse rate, and it is best for patients to discuss these with their doctor to get a more precise estimate of probability.

97. What should I do about routine immunizations? Should I still get a flu shot every year?

After treatment for leukemia with standard chemotherapy, it is not necessary to be reimmunized for childhood illnesses. Of course, you still need to keep up with your tetanus shots, which should be given every 10 years, and an annual flu shot is recommended for adults. In addition, you should have the pneumonia vaccine every 3 years. Special considerations exist for patients who undergo blood or marrow stem cell transplantation. Reimmunization against tetanus, diphtheria, pertussis, hepatitis B, polio, haemophilus influenza type B, pneumococcal pneumonia, and measles-mumps-rubella might be recommended after you are off immunosuppressive drugs. Consult your oncologist before getting immunized, especially if you are not in remission or you are taking immunosuppressive drugs.

Reimmunization against tetanus, diphtheria, pertussis, hepatitis B, polio, haemophilus influenza type B, pneumococcal pneumonia, and measles-mumps-rubella might be recommended after you are off immunosuppressive drugs.

98. What are my legal rights as an employee undergoing treatment and what should I consider if I am looking for a new job?

Like most other serious illnesses, leukemia alters your ability to perform your job. If you are employed, it is wise to seek counsel on what legal protections are available to you in your state. Most states have laws in place that extend your medical insurance for an additional length of time. It is critical for you to keep in contact with your employer's human resources department to be sure that the medical insurance premiums are paid and there is no lapse in coverage.

Most employers are sympathetic to the seriousness of the situation. Knowing the amount of time you are likely to be off and the laws of the state in which you reside, it is wise to be as candid about the situation as is reasonably possible. However, if you do not feel comfortable revealing this information it is not required by law. Employers do not want to lose good employees. It is in their best interest to do all that is necessary to help you win this fight. Depending on what type of job you have and what your treatment is, it is not uncommon to be off the job from several months to more than a year. If your position is physical or requires public contact, then this will be more difficult. Some patients with office or sales positions can telecommute, which is desirable because much of the recovery is slow and boring, but not always that taxing.

If you're looking for a new job, make sure to request information about the company's health benefits when going into an interview. Also ask how long it will take upon hire for the medical coverage to start. Many companies do not start medical coverage until a month or 90 days after hire. Speak to a social worker and ensure that your doctor's visits and treatment are covered. Most medical facilities have an insurance specialist who can help you navigate and understand health insurance policies. Look ahead; make sure the policy will cover a transplant or other treatment that might become necessary. From your current employer, find out about COBRA coverage (what is covered and how long coverage lasts) and what the premiums are. Also determine what paperwork is necessary to sign up.

99. What about the cost and insurance coverage for treatment?

Anyone with leukemia will need to spend time communicating with his or her insurance carrier, because the medical costs are significant and can be catastrophic if not handled well. In most cases, the hospital or physician's office is the mediator with the insurance company as they seek authorization for the proposed treatment plan. Insurance companies almost always consider leukemia a covered illness, but the treatments they cover might not be fully paid. There also can be differences between payment of outpatient versus inpatient treatments. Those who have health maintenance organization coverage should keep the treatment within network facilities, because treatment there is usually covered at a higher percentage than at out-of-network facilities. Patients should contact their insurance company or ask a patient representative at their doctor's office to determine what coverage is available.

The insurance carrier will send an **explanation of benefits** (EOBs). These statements explain the amount of the invoice, what the contract price is, and what they will pay. Most of the time, they also advise patients about what their financial obligation will be. Patients should *not* pay any invoices that are covered by insurance without first receiving their copy of the EOB. It is estimated that up to 80% of medical invoices charged to patients have errors. The caregiver should monitor all procedures and document them.

New treatments and tests are constantly being developed. Insurance companies are not always quick to cover these tests or treatments. If an insurance company does not cover a certain type of treatment there are methods in place to appeal the insurance company's policy. This is especially true if the treatment is absolutely necessary. Patients should remember to always appeal any decision the insurance company makes that is not in the patient's favor. It never hurts to consult the companies producing the treatment as well as nonprofit agencies for assistance. For example, Novartis has an assistance program in place for CML patients whose insurance does not cover imatinib mesylate.

100. Where can I get more information about leukemia?

The information in this book just scratches the surface of what's available to leukemia patients and their families. The Appendix offers a selection of good resources to address many topics. Numerous pamphlets and handouts are also provided by medical institutions so that potential patients can discuss all options available. Be sure to ask for these handouts and any others as they become available. The outpatient clinic where patients receive treatment is a good source for up-to-date information via flyers, posters, and handouts.

Many web sites contain information helpful to patients and physicians. One of the most relevant is that of the Leukemia & Lymphoma Society of America (web site: *www.lls.org*). The Center for International Blood and Marrow Transplant Research (CIBMTR) (web site: *www.cibmtr.org*) posts summary results of hematopoietic stem cell transplantation listed by diseases and **staging** (the extent of the disease), as well as results of autologous versus allogeneic transplantation. The National Marrow Donor Program (NMDP) (web site: *www .marrow.org*) lists the requirements of becoming a hematopoietic stem cell donor and information for potential donors. The American Society of Hematology (ASH) (web site: *www. hematology.org*) is another organization that has helpful education material. The American Association of Blood Banks (AABB) (web site: *www.aabb.org*) provides information about becoming a blood component donor and current tests that are performed on each unit of blood to minimize diseases associated with transfusion. The Foundation for the Accreditation of Cellular Therapy (FACT) (web site: *www.factwebsite.org*) is an organization that produces standards for hematopoietic stem cell transplantation, inspects transplantation centers, and accredits those programs that have met their stringent criteria. The Children's Leukemia Research Association (also called the National Leukemia Research Association) has a web site that appears to address only children's illnesses, yet information on adult leukemia is presented here as well because the web site (*www.childrensleukemia.org*) has expanded. Many nurses belong to the Oncology Nursing Society (ONS), whose web site is at *www.ons.org*. Information about other considerations is found at the Cancer Support Community's web site at *www .cancer-support.org*. Spouses seeking support and information can review material at *www.wellspouse.org*, operated by the Well Spouse Association.

Staging

Evaluating the extent of the disease.

Other academic societies and organizations associated with leukemia that frequently post important and relevant information on their web sites include the American Society of Clinical Oncology (ASCO) (web site: *www.asco.org*) and the Society for Hematology and Stem Cells (ISEH) (web site: *www.iseh.org*). In addition, you might wish to visit the web site of your local healthcare providers, such as major hospitals and cancer centers.

Glossary

A

Acute: Occurring suddenly in a short period of time.

Acute lymphocytic leukemia: Rapidly growing leukemia affecting mature lymphocytes.

Acute myeloid leukemia: Rapidly growing leukemia affecting mature white cells.

Advance directives: Legal documents spelling out how you want your treatment to proceed, including living wills, DNR orders, and durable power of attorney.

ALL: See acute lymphocytic leukemia.

Allogeneic bone marrow transplantation: Bone marrow transplantation using marrow from another person's body.

Allogeneic stem cell transplantation: Cells from another's body are used to treat a cancer.

All-trans-retinoic acid: A drug related to vitamin A that is able to make certain leukemia cells change from blasts to normal mature cells.

Alopecia: Hair loss.

Alternative medicine: Nontraditional medical supplements or techniques.

AML: See acute myeloid leukemia.

Analgesic: Medicine given to control pain.

Anesthesia: Medication that causes entire or partial loss of feeling or sensation.

Antibody: Any of the body's immunoglobulins that are produced in response to specific antigens.

Antiemetic: Medicine that prevents or relieves nausea and vomiting, used during and sometimes after chemotherapy.

Antigen: Substance capable of stimulating an immune response.

Antisense therapy: Emerging investigational therapy for various diseases that blocks protein production.

Apheresis: The process of having peripheral blood stem cells collected.

Aspirate: Removing fluid or cells from tissue by inserting a needle and drawing the fluid into the syringe.

Asymptomatic: Without obvious signs or symptoms of disease.

Attending physician: A fully licensed and board-certified/eligible physician who is on the faculty of the institution or the medical staff.

ATRA: See all-trans-retinoic acid.

Atypical cells: Not usual; abnormal. Cancer is the result of atypical cell division.

Autoimmune process: A reaction of a person's immune system against tissues in his or her own body.

Autologous: Coming from the same person.

Autologous stem cell transplantation: Cells from the patient's own body are used to treat cancer.

B

Biopsy: Surgical removal of a small piece of tissue or a small tumor for microscopic examination to determine whether cancer cells are present. A biopsy is the most important procedure in diagnosing cancer.

Blast: An immature white blood cell that normally represents an early phase of the normal differentiation process that occurs in the bone marrow.

Blast crisis: The evolution of CML in the chronic phase to an acute and aggressive leukemia much like AML.

Blood count: A test to measure the number of red blood cells, white blood cells, and platelets in a blood sample.

Blood transfusion: Replenishment of red blood cells in the bloodstream when one's own bone marrow is unable to do so.

Bone marrow: The soft, fatty substance filling the cavities of the bones. Blood cells are made here.

Bone marrow biopsy/aspiration: A procedure in which a needle is inserted into the center of a bone, usually the hip, to remove a small amount of bone marrow for microscopic examination.

Bone marrow harvest: Under general anesthesia, marrow is collected for later infusion into the patient.

Bone marrow transplant: A procedure in which the bone marrow of a leukemia patient is replaced by another person's marrow.

B lymphocytes: Subset of lymphocytes that make antibodies.

C

Cancer: A general term that describes over 100 different uncontrolled growths of abnormal cells in the body. Cancer cells have the ability to continue to grow, invade, and destroy surrounding tissue.

Cancer cell: A cell that divides and reproduces abnormally with uncontrolled growth. If this cell breaks away and travels to other parts of the body, it is referred to as metastasis.

Carcinogen: Any substance that initiates or promotes the development of cancer.

Caregiver: Acts for the benefit of a patient at the time of serious illness or disease, on the patient's behalf, and assists the patient in making decisions and choices.

Catheter, indwelling: Device placed surgically beneath the skin to facilitate the frequent infusion of medications and/or other treatments (see port-a-cath).

CBC: See complete blood count.

Cell: The basic structural unit of all life. All living matter is composed of cells.

Chemotherapy: Treatment of cancer by use of chemicals; often uses two or more chemicals to achieve maximum kill of tumor cells. Usually refers to drugs used to treat cancer.

Chronic lymphocytic leukemia: A slow-growing leukemia that affects mature lymphocytes.

Chronic: Occurring more slowly and present less dramatically than acute conditions.

Chronic myeloid leukemia: A slow-growing leukemia of mature white blood cells, associated with the Philadelphia chromosome.

Clinical trial: A specific treatment protocol that is designed to test the effectiveness and safety of a drug or combination of drugs, or other therapies, in the treatment of a disease.

Chromosomes: Large complex structures that contain DNA and proteins.

CLL: See chronic lymphocytic leukemia.

CML: See chronic myeloid leukemia.

CMV: See cytomegalovirus.

COBRA: Consolidated Omnibus Budget Reconciliation Act of 1985; ensures continuation of health coverage offered by insurance companies.

Complete blood count: A laboratory test to determine the number of red blood cells, white blood cells, platelets, hemoglobin, and other components of a blood sample.

Complete remission: Total absence of disease.

Congenital disease: A disease existing at or dating from birth.

Consolidation: Additional chemotherapy after remission, often given in cycles.

Cytogenetic analysis: A procedure whereby cells, taken from either the blood or the bone marrow, are cultured in a specialized laboratory in such a way that the dividing cells are arrested in the middle of their division. The structure of the chromosomes can then be stained and visualized by a microscope.

Cytogenetic remission: Remission defined by the chromosomes in the bone marrow cells returning to normal with no evidence of the Philadelphia chromosome.

Cytomegalovirus: A virus similar to herpes virus, which can cause pneumonia, hepatitis, and gastrointestinal illness.

Cytopenia: Low blood count.

Cytotoxic: Drugs that can kill cancer cells. Usually refers to drugs used in chemotherapy treatments.

D

Differentiation: The process during which the stem cell goes through several stages of development.

Diagnosis: The process of identifying a disease by its characteristic signs, symptoms, and laboratory findings.

DNA: One of two nucleic acids (the other is RNA) found in the nucleus of all cells. DNA contains genetic information on cell growth, division, and cell function.

DNA-damaging agents: Known to be initiators of leukemia, including chemicals (benzene and other solvents), ionizing radiation, and some other organic compounds.

DNR order: See do not resuscitate order.

Donor: One who donates blood stem cells or bone marrow for infusion into a patient.

Do not resuscitate order: A medical order telling the medical staff at the hospital or facility that they should not act to revive you in the event that your heart or brain activity cease.

Durable power of attorney: Allows a specific family member to legally make all your decisions, personal and financial, for you in case you become incapacitated.

E

EOB: See explanation of benefits.

Explanation of benefits: A statement of covered assessments and treatments that is provided by the insurance carrier.

F

Flow cytometry: A test performed on cancerous tissues that shows the aggressiveness of the tumor.

FDA: See Food and Drug Administration.

Fellow: A licensed physician who is still in training.

FMLA: See family leave of absence.

Food and Drug Administration: A federal institution charged with approving and regulating medications, foodstuff, and other products for human consumption.

G

G-CSF: See granulocyte colony-stimulating factor.

Genes: Located in the nucleus of the cell, genes contain hereditary information that is transferred from cell to cell.

Gene therapy: Investigational treatment of disease by the introduction of new genetic material into cells in order to modify their DNA.

Genetic: Refers to the inherited pattern located in genes for certain characteristics.

Gleevec: Oral chemotherapy agent approved for use in patients with CML.

GVHD: See graft-versus-host disease.

Granulocyte: White blood cell with a large number of granules.

Graft-versus-host disease: A condition in which the lymphocytes from a donor's stem cells recognize certain antigens on the recipient (patient) as foreign.

Graft-versus-leukemia effect: Occurs when the donor's lymphocytes attack the patient's leukemia cells directly and help in the eradication of the leukemia.

Granulocyte colony-stimulating factor: Growth factors given to activate production of cells.

Growth factors: Substances that promote the growth of white blood cells.

H

Healthcare proxy: Document that limits the decision-making power to only those decisions about your medical treatment.

Hematopoietic growth factors: Drugs that increase blood cell counts.

Hemoglobin: The protein carried by red blood cells that delivers oxygen to the bodies tissues.

Hematologic remission: Remission defined by the blood counts' return to normal.

Hematologist: A specialist who sees and treats patients with malignancies (and other diseases) of the blood.

Hematopoietic stem cell: Referring to its ability to make all the cellular elements of the blood.

Hematopoietic stem cell transplantation: The process by which new stem cells are introduced into a patient.

HLA: See human leukocyte antigen.

HLA-matched sibling: Compatible sister or brother who is determined by testing to be matched at specific loci.

Human leukocyte antigen: The protein on the surface of all cells that must be matched for bone marrow transplants.

Hyperpigmentation: Darkened patches of skin.

I

Immune system: Complex system by which the body protects itself from outside invaders that are harmful to it.

Immunophenotyping: A laboratory test whereby an area's antigens can be measured on the surface of the leukemia cell.

Immunotherapy: Treatment that stimulates the body's own defense mechanisms to combat diseases such as cancer.

Immunosuppression: Condition of having a lowered resistance to disease. May be a temporary result of lowered white blood cells from chemotherapy administration.

Immunosuppressive therapy: Therapy to decrease the response of the immune system.

Incidence: The rate at which a certain event occurs, e.g., the number of new cases of a specific disease occurring during a certain period.

Induction chemotherapy: The initial phase of treatment using medications.

Informed consent: Process of explanation to the patient of all risks and complications of a procedure or treatment before it is done. Most informed consents are written and signed by the patient or a legal representative

Intensification chemotherapy: Use of additional cancer drugs after remission to eliminate any remaining cancer cells.

Intravenously: Entering the body through a vein.

L

Leukemia: A malignancy of a white blood cell in which there is an abnormal accumulation of white blood cells in the blood and the bone marrow.

Leukocyte: A white blood cell or corpuscle.

Living will: Document outlining what care you want in the event that you become unable to communicate due to coma or heavy sedation.

Lymphocytes: Mobile cells made in the bone marrow and lymphoid tissue that are typical cellular elements of lymph and include cellular mediators of immunity; constitute 20%–30% of leukocytes of normal human blood. Come in two major types: B and T.

M

Macrophage: A cell derived from a monocyte that functions to protect against infection and noxious substances.

Malaise: A condition marked by fatigue and overall poor feeling.

Metastasis: The spread of cancer from one part of the body to another through the lymphatic system or the bloodstream.

Microorganism: An organism of minute, microscopic size.

Molecular remission: Remission defined by analysis of small numbers of cells that indicate that a disease is totally eradicated.

Molecule: The smallest particle of a substance that retains the properties of the substance; composed of one or more atoms.

Monoclonal antibody: Antibody that specifically binds to a particular mol-ecule on the surface of a certain type of leukemia or other cancer.

Monocyte: A type of white blood cell that is transported to tissues, where it turns into a macrophage.

Mucositis: A temporary but painful condition in which the lining of the inside of the mouth breaks down, making eating and swallowing difficult.

Myelodysplastic syndrome: A disease of the bone marrow stem cells in which the normal maturation of blood cells is altered.

N

National Marrow Donor Program: A large registry with millions of potential donors in its files for future stem cell transplants.

NMDP: See National Marrow Donor Program.

Neutropenia: A condition in which the body is depleted of important disease-fighting white blood cells.

Neutropenic diet: A diet that avoids foods that might carry harmful bacteria, such as raw meats or fresh fruits and vegetables.

Neutrophil: The most common granulocyte, a type of white blood cell.

O

Ommaya reservoir: A device inserted into the brain for the removal of fluid or instillation of medication.

Oncologist: A physician who specializes in cancer treatment.

Oncology: The science dealing with the physical, chemical and biologic properties and features of cancer, including causes, the disease process, and therapies.

Orally: Taken by mouth.

P

Palliative treatment: Therapy that relieves symptoms but does not alter the development of the disease. Its primary purpose is to improve the quality of life.

Pathogenesis: The origin and development of a disease.

Patient advocate: An individual who serves the needs of the patient, who may be empowered to act on his or her behalf.

Petechiae: Small red dots on the skin as a result of a very low platelet count.

Pharmaceuticals: Medications that are continuously being developed for future patient care.

Philadelphia chromosome: The abnormal chromosome found in patients with CML.

Platelet: A cell formed by the bone marrow and circulating in the blood that is necessary for blood clotting.

Platelet transfusion: Procedure used in cancer patients to prevent or control bleeding when the number of platelets have decreased.

Port-a-cath: A device surgically implanted under the skin, usually on the chest, that enters a large blood vessel and is used to deliver medication, chemotherapy, and blood products; also is used to obtain blood samples.

Prevalence: The number of people alive with a particular disease at any moment.

Prognosis: A prediction of the course of the disease; the future prospect for the patient.

Prognostic factors: Factors that help to determine the severity of a disease.

Prophylactic treatment: Treatment geared to prevent disease or infection.

Protocol: A schedule of selected drugs and treatment time intervals known to be effective against a certain cancer.

R

Radiation oncologist: A specialist trained in the use of high-energy X-rays to treat cancer.

Radiation therapy: treatment with high-energy X-rays to destroy cancer cells.

Relapse: The reappearance of cancer after a disease-free period.

Red blood cells: Hemoglobin-containing cells that carry oxygen to the tissues.

Remission: Complete or partial disappearance of the signs and symptoms of disease in response to treatment; the period during which a disease is under control.

Risk factors: Anything that increases an individual's chance of getting a disease such as cancer.

S

Secondary cancers: A second site where cancer is found.

Secondary leukemia: A malignancy somewhat more common in patients previously treated with certain types of chemotherapy.

Side effects: Usually describes situations that occur after treatments. For example, hair loss may be a side effect of chemotherapy; fatigue may be a side effect of radiation therapy.

Staging: Evaluating the extent of the disease.

Standard protocol: Treatment generally recognized by the medical community as the standard of care.

Stem cells: A primitive type of cell from which all cells of a given organ or tissue arise.

Stem cell transplant: The process by which new stem cells are infused into a patient.

Subcutaneously: Injected under the skin.

Supportive treatment: Treatment with the goal of preserving the strength of the patient.

T

TBI: See total body irradiation.

T lymphocytes: Lymphocytes that directly attach themselves to virally infected or transformed cells to mediate their destruction.

Tissue: A collection of similar cells. There are four basic types of tissues in the body: epithelial, connective, muscle, and nerve.

Total body irradiation: Treatment in which the entire body is exposed to the same intensity of radiation, which is precisely determined by the radiation oncologist to remove all indication of disease.

Translocation: The movement of one piece of chromosome to another chromosome.

Trisomy 12: An extra chromosome 12 that is frequently present in patients with CLL.

Tumor: An abnormal tissue, swelling, or mass; may be either benign or malignant.

Venoocclusive disease: A sometimes fatal condition that can lead to liver failure; requires rapid medical intervention.

W

WBC: See white blood cell.

White blood cell: Blood cells that do not contain hemoglobin; also called leukocytes.

Appendix

American Association of Blood Banks (AABB)

8101 Glenbrook Road
Bethesda, MD 20814
Phone: 301-907-6977
Web site: *www.aabb.org*

This site provides information about becoming a blood component donor and current tests that are performed on each unit of blood to minimize diseases associated with transfusion.

American Cancer Society (ACS)

1599 Clifton Road NE
Atlanta, GA 30329
Phone: 800-ACS-2345
Web site: *www.cancer.org*

American Society of Clinical Oncology (ASCO)

2318 Mill Road, Suite 800
Alexandria, VA 22314
Phone: 571-483-1300
Web site: *www.asco.org*

American Society of Hematology (ASH)

2021 L Street NW, Suite 900
Washington, DC 20036
Phone: 202-776-0544
Web site: *www.hematology.org*

Blood & Marrow Transplant Information Network

2310 Skokie Valley Road, Suite 104
Highland Park, IL 60035
Phone: 888-597-7674 or
847-433-3313
Web site: *www.bmtinfonet.org*

The Bone Marrow Foundation

30 East End Avenue, Suite 1F
New York, NY 10028
Phone: 212-838-3029 or
800-365-1336
Web site: *www.bonemarrow.org*

CancerCare

275 Seventh Avenue, Floor 22
New York, NY 10001
Phone: 800-813-HOPE (4673)
Web site: *www.CancerCare.org*

Cancer Support Community

4918 Cooper Road
Cincinnati, OH 45242
Phone: 513-791-4060
Web site: *www.cancer-support.org*

Center for International Blood and Marrow Transplant Research (CIBMTR)

Froedtert and the Medical College of Wisconsin Clinical Cancer Center

9200 W. Wisconsin Avenue, Suite C5500
Milwaukee, WI 53226
Phone: 414-805-0700
Web site: *www.cibmtr.org*

Children's Leukemia Research Association

585 Stewart Avenue, Suite 18
Garden City, NY 11530
Phone: 516-222-1944
Web site: *www.childrensleukemia.org*

While the site states only "children's leukemia," there is information on adult leukemia as well.

The Foundation for the Accreditation of Cellular Therapy (FACT)

986065 Nebraska Medical Center
Omaha, NE 68198
Phone: 402-559-1950
Web site: *www.factwebsite.org*

This organization produces standards for hematopoietic stem cell transplantation, inspects transplantation centers, and accredits those programs that have met its stringent criteria.

The International Bone Marrow Transplant Registry (IBMTR)

See Center for International Blood and Marrow Transplant Research (CIBMTR).

Leukemia & Lymphoma Society

1311 Mamaroneck Avenue, Suite 310
White Plains, NY 10605
Phone: 800-955-4572
Call for local chapter information.
Web site: *www.lls.org*

National Cancer Institute (NCI)

NCI Public Inquiries Office
6116 Executive Boulevard, Suite 300
Bethesda, MD 20892-8322
Phone: 800-4-CANCER
Web site: *www.cancer.gov*

National Leukemia Research Association

See Children's Leukemia Research Association.

National Marrow Donor Program (NMDP)

3001 Broadway Street NE, Suite 100
Minneapolis, MN 55413-1753
Phone: 800-MARROW2
Web site: *www.marrow.org*

This site lists the requirements of becoming a hematopoietic stem cell donor and information for potential donors.

Oncology Nursing Society (ONS)

125 Enterprise Drive
Pittsburgh, PA 15275
Phone: 866-257-4ONS
Web site: *www.ons.org*

Society for Hematology and Stem Cells (ISEH)

401 N. Michigan Avenue, Suite 2200
Chicago, IL 60611
Phone: 312-321-5114
Web site: *www.iseh.org*

Well Spouse Association

63 West Main Street, Suite H
Freehold, NJ 07728
Phone: 800-838-0879
Web site: *www.wellspouse.org*

Index

side effects of, 53

Cytarabine. *See* Cytosine arabinoside

Cytogenetic analysis, 17, 27–30

Cytokines, 34, 41

Cytomegalovirus (CMV), 69

Cytopenia, definition of, 16

Cytosar-U. *See* Cytosine arabinoside

Cytosine arabinoside
  for acute myeloid leukemia, 12
  trade and slang names of, 35

Cytotoxic, definition of, 34

Cytotoxic drugs, 34, 65–66

Dacogen (decitabine), 16, 44

Dasatinib (Sprycel), 12, 14, 29, 36
  for acute lymphoblastic leukemia,
    36
  for chronic myeloid leukemia, 14,
    36

Death/dying
  acceptance of, 86
  legal steps in, 90–92
  preparation for, 88–90

Decitabine, 16, 44

Development of drugs, 36, 43–44

Dexamethasone, for
    immunosuppression in transplant,
    53

Diagnosis, definition of, 16

Diet, 21–22, 25, 66–67

Dietary supplements, 63–64

Differentiation
  definition of, 6
  stem cell, 5–6

DNA, 28, 39

DNA damage, 6–7

DNR order, 88, 90, 91

Doctors
  attending *versus* fellow, 75–76
  evaluation of, 74–75

Donors, stem cell, 49–51, 55–57
  age of, 57–58
  contact with, 56
  definition of, 49
  HLA testing of, 57
  registry/sources of, 56–57
  related, 49–50, 57
  sibling, 49–50, 57
  time to acquire, 55–56
  unrelated, 50, 56

Do not resuscitate (DNR) order, 88,
    90

Down syndrome, and leukemia, 7, 20
  definition of, 90

Drug(s). *See also* Chemotherapy;
    specific agents
  commonly used, *11*
  cytotoxic, 34, 65–66
  in development, 36, 43–44
  study, 43–44

Drug names, 35

Durable powers of attorney, 90

Eating, 21–22, 25, 66–67

Electrical power lines, and leukemia, 7

Eligibility for clinical trials, 44–45

Employment
  and health care insurance, 86–88
  leave of absence from, 86–88
  legal rights in, 100–101
  return to, 97

End-of-life decisions and care, 88–90

Eosinophils, *4*

Erythropoietin, for myelodysplastic
    syndrome, 16

Exercise, 22, 98

Explanation of benefits (EOBs), 102

Family history, 19–20

Family Medical Leave Act (FMLA),
    86–87